Let's talk about your new family's sleep

Let's talk about your new family's sleep

Lyndsey Hookway

Let's talk about your new family's sleep

First published in the UK by Pinter & Martin Ltd 2020
Reprinted 2021

Copyright © Lyndsey Hookway 2020

All rights reserved

ISBN 978-1-78066-705-8

Also available as an ebook

The right of Lyndsey Hookway to be identified as the author of this work has been asserted by her in accordance with the Copyright, Designs and Patent Act of 1988

Edited by Susan Last
Index by Helen Bilton
Design by Blok Graphic

British Library Cataloguing-in-Publication Data
A catalogue record for this book is available from the British Library

Printed in the EU by Hussar

This book has been printed on paper that is sourced and harvested from sustainable forests and is FSC accredited
Pinter & Martin Ltd
6 Effra Parade
London SW2 1PS

pinterandmartin.com

Contents

Introduction

Welcome to the world of sleep! You might be a new parent. You might have literally just seen two blue lines on a pregnancy test and you're already thinking about how you'll cope with sleep deprivation. Have you heard horror stories about sleep? Conflicting opinions about the best way to handle night waking? Maybe you've been handed various books and you've been promised that 'this one is the only book you'll need'? Or perhaps you're already knee deep in baby toys and laundry and trying to figure out how to navigate the great sleep confusion.

However you ended up with this book in your hands – congratulations. You're about to see sleep in a new and positive way, that doesn't need to feel like a mission. Sleep, like many other areas of parenting, is emotionally charged and fraught with controversy, but this book is here to ease the stress and make sleep a normal and positive part of gentle parenting.

I don't know who first uttered the phrase 'sleep like a baby'. You've heard it, you might even have said it a few times. But when you stop to think about what it means, it's pretty obvious that whoever said it in the first place probably wasn't referring to sleeping solidly all night.

I wonder if what they meant was that when babies are sleeping, they seem to sleep in sweet contentment. Many babies can sleep in cars, while being moved around, or with background noise. I wish I could sleep like that! Have you ever watched a baby sleeping? Really watched them? Ever consciously thought about the effect that being near a peacefully sleeping baby has on you? For many, it is impossible not to be positively affected by the experience of holding a sleeping baby close, staring into their face, wondering what they dream about, and feeling the contagious relaxing effects of their carefree slumber.

What if parents could be just as relaxed about sleep as babies are? Wouldn't that be great? I wonder what parenting would feel like if it didn't feel like a competition. Whose offspring can sleep the longest, the earliest, the most predictably? What if we could embrace sleep as another part of responsive parenting?

This is not another book telling you how to raise your baby, promising you a certain amount of sleep in a certain number of days or weeks. This book will not tell you how to get your baby sleeping through the night, or provide you with a step-by-step guide to naps, or bedtime routines. What it will do is support you to feel calm, confident and connected in your parenting. It will encourage you to choose to listen to your gut instinct, and ignore those who claim that the only way to get some sleep is to leave your baby to cry.

The truth is, sleep does not need to feel like a battleground. You are not fighting a sleep war, and your baby is not a sleep thief! Sadly, too many people try to measure their 'success' as a parent by objective and quantifiable parameters like how much and how 'well' their baby sleeps.

I've been supporting families with sleep for many years. Usually within the first 10 minutes of a conversation with a parent they have told me that they feel guilty about their child's sleep. They admit that they feel the way their child sleeps is their fault, or that they are failing their baby in some way. Dear parent, if you feel this way, I want you to know right now that it is not your job to make your child sleep. You cannot force it. You have not messed up. You are enough for your child.

The reason I know that you need to hear that is that back

" The truth is, sleep does not need to feel like a battleground. You are not fighting a sleep war, and your baby is not a sleep thief!"

in 2009 I needed to hear it too. I was a professional mum with a background in children's nursing and health visiting and I assumed that my training would equip me to have sleep nailed. Oh, how wrong I was! Both of my beautiful girls have taught me a huge amount about sleep. About not getting sleep. How it feels emotionally to be sleep deprived, or feel not good enough. How it feels when it seems the whole world has got sleep figured out and your baby is the only one still waking every hour all night. How it feels when nearly everyone, including health professionals, friends, family and colleagues, is telling you that you just need to leave your baby to cry. The sense of desperation when you know that leaving your baby to cry is not what you want to do, yet you feel utterly broken and desperate and have actually wondered whether you can die from lack of sleep.

It sometimes felt to me that there was nothing that fit my situation. There was plenty of advice to leave my baby to cry, or put her on a schedule, stop night feeds, or just stop breastfeeding. There was also a lot of information that seemed to be telling me that it was all normal, that it was a phase, and that it would pass. None of this worked for me. I was not coping, I was overwhelmed and although I knew it would probably improve in time, I really needed an improvement soon. The last 10 years for me have been a deep dive into the world of sleep, with a specific focus on the parents who, like me, don't want to leave their babies to cry, but also need some sensible and practical solutions.

I know from both personal experience and from supporting parents over the years, that it is easy for sleep to become an obsession. I liken the obsession to needing to use the bathroom – stick with me on this! Have you ever been driving in a car, and just as you pass a service station it suddenly occurs to you that you are actually quite desperate for the bathroom? You then can't think of anything except how badly you need to go, and you wish you had stopped when you had the chance. You begin to wonder when there will be another service station. Should you pull over? Is it legal to go to the bathroom by the side of the highway? Every noise sounds like a waterfall. You're acutely aware of the drinks bottles littering the car – the fluids that have directly contributed to the urgent sensation in your bladder. You wonder if you could 'go' in one of those bottles... In fact, you can't really think of anything except how much you need to go. Sleep can feel like this as well. You wake up tired, wondering when you'll next have an opportunity to sleep. You pray to anyone who might be listening that the baby will nap so that you can too. You dread a refused nap because you don't know how you can go on without some sleep. You begin to wish crazy things – like someone will miraculously come over and entertain the baby while you go back to bed, or your partner will come home from work early (even though that has literally never happened) so you can get to sleep. You entertain fantasies of going to a fancy hotel for a week and just sleeping. You google sleep. You talk about sleep. You think about sleep. All the time. But did you know: this is likely to make you feel worse. The more we obsess over sleep, the worse it often gets, and the worse we tend to feel about it. The more we worry about sleep, over-think it, and dread it, the worse it usually gets. The opposite is also true, thankfully! This means that if you can learn to take the pressure off yourself and your baby, the better you'll cope. The more positively you feel about sleep, the more relaxed you can learn to be, and the less stressful sleep feels. Changing the way we feel about sleep is crucial to sleep success.

Realistic expectations about sleep take the pressure off the need for you – the parent – to achieve a particular sleep outcome. But more than that, giving sleep its proper position in the landscape of parenting avoids an over-emphasis on sleep above everything else – such as attachment, fun, feeding, relationships, and figuring out family time, as well as making sure that emotional health and wellbeing and a healthy lifestyle are important parts of life. When we learn to get this balance, sleep often falls into place. We feel more confident, and we stop feeling like we are failing, and start believing that we are enough.

I don't promise to know all the answers, or to have the magic wand I know everyone is still looking for. Parenting is hard even when you get plenty of sleep, and I can't and don't want to minimise the effort of the important work you are doing with your child. I just want to see a world where babies are not punished for sleeping like babies – which, as we know, is a bit of a confusing sentiment in the first place.

Chapter one

Addressing sleep myths

→ What's the craziest thing you've been told will help your baby sleep? I've heard some strange ideas over the years. Some of them make me laugh, some make me angry, some are downright weird. Mostly, myths about sleep make me sad. This is because when parents are desperate for sleep, especially if they don't have a lot of support, they are sometimes willing to try anything, even if they don't naturally feel drawn to that particular strategy.[1] Telling people to try something that ultimately will probably not work is misleading, unethical and risks you feeling a failure, when actually the advice was just dumb to start with.

Sleep myths often *sound* like they might be sensible – so it can be hard to tell the myths from the truth. After all, who really has time to go through all the blogs and articles, books and videos about sleep and classify them into 'true', 'false', 'unhelpful', and 'totally off the wall'. Especially if you're sleep-deprived, some of the well-written advice you read or hear about can sound compassionate, supportive or even clever.

I'm going to explain 10 of the most prevalent myths you'll come across, where these myths come from, why people think they work, and why, in fact, they do not work. Consider this your cut-out-and-stick-on-the-fridge list of things not to listen to the next time someone suggests one. You get an extra virtual hug if you're unlucky enough to have every single one of these suggestions thrown your way.

Myth #1: Give the baby a bottle

I expect nearly every parent has heard a variation on this. It may be that you have been advised to top up after a bedtime breastfeed, give a larger volume of milk before bed if you're formula feeding, or offer expressed milk in a bottle rather than breastfeed. None of this advice is based on evidence. There will always be someone who claims that one of these strategies was the miracle cure for their baby's sleep, but in general, large studies have not found that this will make a huge difference to the way your baby sleeps.[2]

It sounds sensible on one level, doesn't it – after all, if your car has an empty tank of petrol, it can't run very far. You fill it up, and it can go further. Except that this isn't quite how it works with babies. A car uses up fuel as it runs, in quite a consistent fashion. If you drive for 500 miles, you will steadily use up fuel. However, with human digestion, how quickly you empty your stomach isn't entirely dependent on how much you consume in one go.[3] Babies can't store up 'fuel' to keep themselves going for extra time. It would be nice if they could! But it just doesn't make sense. Actually, some research has shown that the opposite is true, and that the larger the feed volume, the faster the stomach will empty.[4]

Another thing to remember is that breastfed babies drink approximately the same amount of milk over a 24-hour period between the ages of 1–6 months.[5] This means that if they suddenly start feeding more often, it has nothing to do with trying to *increase* your milk supply, as many people still believe, and everything to do with the fact that for one reason or another – usually developmental – they need to breastfeed more often.[6] They will probably drink less at each feed if they feed often, and again, some research suggests that this is to do with the changing milk composition, faster stomach emptying time, or an increased need for comfort.[7] But whatever the reason, it's important to know this, because if the total daily milk volume stays about the same, then giving extra milk in the assumption that your baby is *extra* hungry will not work.

Sometimes the advice to give a bottle stems from the idea that a bottle might be less soothing and more restrictive than breastfeeding.[8] This particular theory is not research-based in the slightest, and I have seen plenty of babies who fall asleep on a bottle as readily as they do on the breast. Of course, giving a baby a bottle means that someone else can

"Too often we end up getting the message that the only reasonable excuse for waking up at night is because of a genuine need for food, and that all other reasons are unnecessary."

feed them, but you'll need to make sure that firstly you don't become uncomfortably engorged, and secondly that you will actually be able to sleep. The slightly maddening thing that many parents find is that when given the opportunity to sleep, they can't because they are worrying about their baby.[9] So make sure you can totally trust the person who will feed and look after your baby if you do decide to try this to catch up on some sleep. Also, don't forget that it is not all-or-nothing. You can try this as a temporary measure, and then abandon it if you don't like it or find it helpful.

The other problem is that if you over-feed a baby, not only can this have a negative effect on your milk supply if you're breastfeeding, but it can also stretch your baby's tummy and leave them feeling stuffed or uncomfortable.[10] If you over-eat, you tend to want to go to sleep, but if you keep doing this, your appetite will increase overall as your stomach stretches. The same can happen with a baby. I've worked with countless parents who have tried this strategy, and the story they tell me is nearly always the same – it didn't stop their baby waking up, and often it made them wake up even hungrier for the next night feed.

The final problem with this advice is that it implies that babies wake up at night primarily due to hunger, and that feeding at night is only about meeting this need for food. The truth is that babies wake up for many reasons, and while feeding them at night may help them go back to sleep, the feed does not necessarily meet a need relating to hunger. They may have woken for another important reason – such as warmth, connection, and comfort. Too often we end up getting the message that the only reasonable excuse for waking up at night is because of a genuine need for food, and that all other reasons are unnecessary. But as you're probably aware, even you and I wake up at night for random reasons from time to time.

Myth #2: Only feed every four hours

This is still a very prevalent piece of advice. If you think about it, it's a close relative of myth #1. It comes from the same idea that babies only wake up due to hunger, so making sure that they're not 'just feeding for comfort' will make them sleep. This is simply not true, and does babies a great disservice.

If we apply a little logic here, there are a couple of reasons why people might think this would work:

1. The baby is feeding for comfort, and this is unnecessary
2. The baby must be taught to only feed when they are actually hungry

If the baby is actually hungry, then feeding them less often isn't going to work, because they will just be hungry and will cry more or wake more due to hunger. If they are not hungry, but feeding for comfort, then the parent will have to find another way of comforting them, because the need for comfort isn't going to go away. Sure, you can ignore that need, but we'll come back to why that might not be such a great idea later on.

Furthermore, some babies have very small appetites. If you feed them less often, you risk them not being able to get enough calories during a 24-hour period. If they are bottle-fed, this may stretch their tummy – which may have a detrimental impact on their appetite regulation later on. If breastfed, this strategy is risky because it assumes that breasts always make the same amount of milk each time (they don't), and that you can control how much milk a baby drinks in one feed (you can't), and that the mother can store that larger amount of milk necessary for less frequent feeds (not always possible).

Finally, as I mentioned before, babies feed frequently for many reasons. Just because they may settle after a feed, doesn't mean that hunger was why it was appropriate to feed them. I know that might take some getting your head around, but feeding and hunger are not always the same thing. We've come to think about this with an adult mentality of equating comfort-feeding with over-eating. But while eating too much food as an adult is not a good idea, it's not really a principle that can be applied to young breastfed infants, as there are many complex (and really quite clever) mechanisms to regulate and control milk intake and appetite in a breastfed baby. It is more possible to over-feed a formula-fed baby, but as long as you keep an eye on the total daily volume, you still don't need to worry too much.

Myth #3: By x weeks/months/x amount of weight, your baby should be sleeping x hours solid at night

Many people who hold tight to this advice don't realise that the paper they may be unwittingly referring to dates back to the 1950s. That's not exactly up-to-date research! This is probably the most widely circulated myth, and is often to be found in combination with another one – for example, the belief that your baby will sleep through the night once they also are on solids at six months. Or that they will sleep through when they are on four-hourly feeds by four months. I also frequently hear that when a baby weighs a certain amount, or has doubled their birth weight, they will sleep – the list of random associations goes on. Whether this is a stand-alone statement or in conjunction with another myth – it is still a myth. I've met many babies who sleep through the night from an early age, and I meet many more who are still waking at night into their third year of life and beyond. It really is individual, highly variable and multi-factorial. Again, there will always be a baby in your circle of friends who fits the mould, but your baby is unique – don't fall in to the trap of comparing.

Myth #4: Start solids

There has actually been a reasonable amount of research on this topic in recent years, and some research studies disagree.[11,12] The main reason people believe that starting solids will help is closely related to the reason behind myths #1 and #2: hunger. The theory is that if the baby is waking excessively at night due to hunger, giving them a square meal will sort the problem out. That would be a nice, tidy theory, if firstly they were only waking due to hunger, and secondly they could eat enough calories to store up overnight to get them through – which, as we discovered with myth #1, is not true. The other problem is that the type of foods we tend to give babies who are just getting started with solids are not calorie dense. What might be a good first food? Steamed carrot batons perhaps? Some ripe pear wedges? Given the size of a baby's tummy, they won't be able to fit a whole banana in! They will probably manage to eat a carrot baton or two, and spit half of it out. That's maybe five calories. There is nothing more nutrient-dense than milk at this age. So the reality is that even if a baby were waking at night due to hunger (which we have established is not the whole story), giving them solids is unlikely to help – in fact, it may deny them calories! Solids are really important, at the right time, but we should be careful not to expect miracles from them. At the present time, the research we have available suggests that starting solids early will not help, and there are no associated health benefits of starting solids early anyway – so it cannot be justified.

Myth #5: Stop breastfeeding

This is still a common idea, based on some research showing that in the very early days formula-fed babies seem to last a little longer between feeds. It's not hugely significant – perhaps one less wake-up at night for the formula-fed infants.[13,14] But these differences disappear after about the age of four months, with both breast and formula-feeding babies waking equally often.[15] Even when parents feed their babies more frequently in the day and reduce feeds at night, it doesn't seem to reduce the number of night *wake-ups* – just the number of night *feeds*. Reading between the lines, what this means is that if you bottle-feed, you still have to get up, but you just find other ways of getting your baby to fall asleep again that do not involve feeding.

There has been some really interesting recent research that compared parent reports of how much babies were sleeping with results from a special device used to measure sleep scientifically, called an actigraph. For years, sleep research has assumed that parent reports of how much babies are sleeping are accurate. But this research found that the breastfeeding families were *under*estimating their baby's sleep compared to the sleep actigraph, and the formula-feeding families were *over*estimating their babies sleep compared to the actigraph.[16] So – is all the research actually inaccurate anyway? Do we need to go back and repeat every study that's ever compared the ways in which breast and formula-fed babies sleep, when it relies on parental report? I don't know. But it should certainly make us question the data.

Breastfeeding is known to be of fantastic benefit to both babies and mothers, and if you're enjoying it, and your baby is thriving, then don't let sleep be the thing that sways you to stop. In fact, large research studies have found that breastfeeding parents

" Children learn independence by first having their needs for dependence met. "

get more sleep.[17] I meet so many people who have stopped breastfeeding because they were desperate for sleep, who tell me that it didn't work, and that they are sad they stopped. Of course, breastfeeding is a highly personal decision, and this isn't about forcing anyone to continue. But don't stop for the sake of sleep – that's all I'm saying!

Myth #6: Stop bed-sharing

There are variations on the reasons given for suggesting this one. You might hear that you'll still have a child in your bed when they're 7, 10, 15, or whatever. You might also hear that attachment parenting is to blame, or that it will make your child clingy and dependent on you for longer. The opposite is actually true. Children learn independence by first having their needs for dependence met.[18] Leaving aside any arguments about safety, the cultural variations in opinion and the personal reasons why parents choose to bed-share, let's think about what the research around bed-sharing is actually saying.

Firstly, there is some evidence that sharing a bed is associated with more night waking,[19] but it may be more complicated than it first appears. The thing is that some parents choose to bed-share because they are *already* struggling with sleep – so in fact, bed-sharing could be the response to sleep challenges, not the cause of it.[20]

Other studies find that parents who bed-share get more sleep than those who don't. This could be because when babies or children are in the same bed, their parent does not need to get up and resettle their child – nearly all children go to sleep more easily and quickly when in bed with a parent.[21]

One thing is for sure: no study finds a link between bed-sharing and clingy behaviour or a lack of later independence, so whether you choose to move on from bed-sharing, or not start in the first place, don't let this particular argument sway you.

Myth #7: Move the baby into another room

The idea of minimising nighttime contact, avoiding too much interaction, and having separate bedrooms for babies was first talked about by a well-known American paediatrician called Emmett Holt.[22] He was a firm advocate of crying-it-out and putting babies in separate bedrooms.[23,24] Moving into more recent times, many parenting authors and sleep 'experts' recommend a 'robotic' or minimal interaction response in the night, avoiding eye-contact and not speaking to your child. To *some* extent, they have a point – after all, if we start dancing around or singing, putting the TV on or playing games in the night then this is extremely confusing for a baby who is learning to tell the difference between night and day.

However, there is a big difference between gentle, responsive but quiet care of infants at night, and deliberately avoiding eye-contact with them, and refusing to engage in any way. As with many things, a middle ground interpretation is a good idea.

Keeping your baby in the room with you until at least six months is the current guideline in the UK. In the US, the American Academy of Pediatrics has recently changed its recommendation to 12 months – you can only imagine the debate that particular suggestion has sparked! As for your response to your baby in the night: I suggest you adopt a loving, warm and compassionate approach, while also keeping your interaction low-key, quiet and calm.

Myth #8: Ignore your baby's cries

I doubt whether anyone has *not* heard about leaving a baby to cry in order to teach them to go to sleep with minimal parental intervention. Recent research suggests that this has become embedded in Western culture.[25] The suggestion stems from the idea that crying is a learned behaviour, and parental intervention is a 'reward' for that behaviour. Therefore, responding to the child reinforces and encourages the child to carry on crying in order to get a response from a parent. This theory is called behaviourism, and actually dates back to the early 1900s,[26] though prominent paediatricians have been warning parents not to 'give in' to their baby's demands for fear of 'spoiling' them for at least 200 years. This is definitely not a modern approach to dealing with sleep.

But is it really as simple as this? Do we do babies a disservice by assuming that their cries for a response are not meaningful? I believe that all crying is communication, and all communication is meaningful. Denying a response because of a belief that the reason for the crying is unimportant, unnecessary, or irrelevant sends a confusing message to a child who is not mature enough to understand the fact that crying at night is inconvenient for a tired parent. We surely want our children to know that if they have a problem, they can trust their parent to help them with that problem. Too often, nighttime communication is perceived as problematic, except under specific, adult-driven parameters and expectations. So, for example, a baby crying to be fed may be ignored because 'they can't possibly be hungry'. The misunderstanding of the fact that feeding meets more needs than just nutrients and calories is at the heart of the problem of this interpretation. Furthermore, leaving a child to cry is not the only way to improve sleep.[27]

We will come back to the subject of leaving babies to cry a little later, but for now, I'll leave you with the idea that ignoring crying may eventually teach a child not to expect a response from their parent – but is this what we ultimately want our children to learn?

> **" We surely want our children to know that if they have a problem, they can trust their parent to help them with that problem. "**

Myth #9: You need to put them down drowsy but awake from the beginning

Honestly, who *hasn't* heard this one? If there's one phrase that drives tired parents crazy it's this. The demoralising experience of attempting to comfort a child awake, and then place them in a cot or crib awake, only to have them start crying again has to be one of the most frustrating and stressful parenting moments. I vividly remember feeling utterly per-plexed about why my first baby seemed to have a gravity sensor and the moment I started to lay her flat, she would instantly wake up and start howling. I quickly abandoned it, and all ideas about persevering with it.

The idea comes from the desire to distance a particular activity from a particular outcome – for example, feeding or rocking to sleep.

These actions are often known as sleep associations. In fairness, there is probably a grain of truth in it – after all, we establish habits from repeating patterns of behaviour. But once again, has a general truth been extrapolated too far, and applied to the wrong people or circumstances?

I usually take a pragmatic approach with this. If your baby remains sleepy and is content to be placed in their cot or crib drowsy, then there is nothing wrong with continuing to do this. If, however, your baby becomes upset and wakes up, becoming distressed, then some researchers believe that this can create an association between feeling sleepy and being abruptly woken up.[28] If you think about it, it makes a lot of sense that this is a bad idea from the perspective of creating positive sleep habits.

Other reasons I would recommend ignoring this piece of advice are if you *enjoy* doing whatever it is you do to get your baby to sleep – whether that is holding, rocking, feeding or walking in the baby carrier – or if it becomes stressful for you to persevere. Parenting is a two-way relationship: it is not just about what your baby finds positive and soothing, but also about your feelings and wishes as well.

Myth #10: If you don't teach your baby to sleep well, it's bad for their development

I hear this particular viewpoint from about half of my clients. Many of them are actually more worried about their child's development than their own sleep. They call me and wonder aloud whether they are letting their baby down in terms of future development by not helping them to sleep now. There is certainly a lot of evidence about the impact of sleep deprivation on adults, teenagers and school-age children. The message with these age groups is clear – delaying bedtime and not getting enough sleep has negative impacts on mood, cognitive function and memory. But can we say the same of babies and younger children? Well – the jury is definitely out.

There seems to be an even split of research studies that suggest that lack of sleep and fragmented sleep has a negative impact on later cognitive function,[29-32] but there are equal numbers of studies that find no association between sleep problems in infancy (as defined by the researchers and parents) and later cognitive outcomes.[33-36] So, it seems, looking to science, that we are none the wiser. Again, ever the pragmatist, my feeling is that babies and young children are probably sleeping no differently now than they ever have, so it is probably not sensible to think that their normal sleep patterns are affecting development.

So there you have 10 myths that on the face of it, don't look too ludicrous, but actually, when you wrap your head around them, have very little evidence behind them. The truth is that most parents would probably stand on their head, dance under the light of a full moon or eat bugs if it was suggested as an infant sleep remedy, but the more sensible-sounding suggestions are often just as unlikely as bug-eating to help with sleep. For this reason, the pseudo-sensible myths are more dangerous than the totally crazy suggestions, because they are more likely to be carried out. Trying a suggestion that is not evidence-based is dangerous for a couple of reasons. Firstly, it is unlikely to work, which may cause you to blame yourself or your baby. This is not fair on anyone. You are not failing, and your baby is not broken – it's just a dumb strategy. Secondly, it may make you do something that is not in your or your baby's best interests – such as putting your baby in their own room too soon, stopping doing something that you love, or starting solids too soon, which may be bad for your baby's health and development.

Chapter two

The truth about sleep

→ Having laughed, sighed and cried over the myths that may have led you up the sleep garden path, I now want to stop talking about things that are untrue, and concentrate on what is true.

Many parents are trying to raise children in a society that still does not fully value the worth of parenting. Even you may not realise your own worth as a parent, surrounded as you probably are by a minefield of opinions, judgements and comments about how you choose to raise your children. You may have worked or studied before you started a family, or you may not. Either way, adjusting to the role of being the sole provider and role model for tiny humans is an enormous responsibility that you likely had no training for, no annual appraisal to discuss your next goal, or a pay rise to acknowledge the hard work you put in. You pour your heart and soul into being a mum, or dad, or whatever parenting title you choose to adopt, and yet very few people sit you down and tell you you're doing a good job. Perhaps this is because parenting is not technically a 'job' – it is a relationship. But it is a unique relationship, and probably the most profound one you will ever experience. To undertake this relationship effectively, you need to know what your role is, and what you can let go of.

Truth #1: The measure of how 'good' a parent you are is not how 'well' your child sleeps

I cannot stress this enough. In many areas of life, success is measured by outcomes, objectives and quantifiable facts. In parenting, there is very little objective and quantifiable feedback to reassure you that you are doing well. Sometimes our human nature means that we seem to be drawn towards looking for things that we can measure. The only objective pieces of data in parenting are how well your child feeds and sleeps. Therefore, a temptation exists for you, or others around you, to measure parenting success on these outcomes. For example, the number of hours your child sleeps, whether they sleep through the night, how few night feeds you do, or whether they are putting on weight.

If only we could measure our effort rather than the outcome we might feel better about it! If only we could measure the impact of all that lovely gentle responsive parenting on later security, confidence and empathy. But sadly we can't – at least not right now, when you need it, and not in a way that gives you immediate feedback. The other truth bomb is that some children are easier-going than others. Often, even within families, one sibling is easier-going than the other. If the Universe is playing a cruel joke, you may get two children who test your parenting skills – or maybe Mother Nature just knows you're the best person for the job!

I remember going to coffee shops with my eldest who simply wouldn't sleep in the day unless she was rocked in a very specific way. I used to almost *hate* my friends whose babies just lay gurgling in their pushchairs while mine was on high alert the whole time. The sidelong glances as I tried to distract my shrieking baby used to make me feel two inches tall. Worse still was when they hinted that their baby's contentment was due to the routine they had implemented so successfully. I knew this wasn't true even then, but now, thankfully, we have scientific evidence to back this up. Strict routines only work for about 15–20% of all babies[1] – and these little ones probably would have gravitated towards this anyway, as it's in their nature.[2] A higher-need baby may require more effort on your part,[3] yet it may feel like the effort you put in does not equate to positive sleep outcomes.

I really want you to know that if this is you, that you are not alone, that you are doing a great job, and you will one day see the fruits of your labours.

" I really want you to know that you are not alone, that you are doing a great job, and you will one day see the fruits of your labours. "

Until then, keep the faith, and read this paragraph as many times as it takes for you to be able to repeat it to yourself as a daily mantra. You are awesome.

Truth #2: Perfect parents do not exist. You are enough for your child

When we envisage parenting before our children come along, we often see visions reminiscent of Mary Poppins, who is endlessly kind, patient, fun, and has total calm authority. Of course, we saw kids losing it in super-markets, or running rings round their exhausted parents who gave in and bought them toys just to buy three minutes' peace... We weren't blind! We just *knew* that wouldn't happen to us! No way would we spawn offspring who disrespect us in public. I think naivety is Nature's way of not putting us off procreation. If we knew what we were letting ourselves in for, it would change the way we anticipate the arrival of our children, wouldn't it?

Anyway, raising children is wonderful. And it is also exhausting, frustrating, bewildering, confusing, annoying and hilarious. There are days when you will hide in the bathroom, and there are days when you want to freeze time. The paradox of parenting is that it is awful and amazing sometimes at exactly the same moment. It's okay if you don't love every minute. It's okay if you feel like you didn't get it all right. Children don't need perfect parents, which is just as well, as they do not exist. You just need to get it right enough of the time. When you get it wrong (because you absolutely will), then model how we make relationships right again by apologising. Being real, authentic and honest with your children will set them up to be emotionally intelligent and resilient little people.

You are almost certainly your own worst critic. Most of us wouldn't dream of being as unkind to others as we are to ourselves. Practise self-compassion and self-forgiveness – it will stop you setting yourself up to fail. We spend a lot of time talking about having realistic expectations of our children, but you also need to have realistic expectations of yourself. You are, after all, only human.

Truth #3: Children do not need to be 'taught' how to sleep

I get really fed up with the idea that babies and children are somehow inept and do not know how to fall asleep. Sleep is not a learned skill, but a homeostatic bodily function. Sure, there are things you can do to encourage and facilitate more sleep, or better sleep, but left to their own devices, every human on the planet will sleep, whether they want to or not. It will simply overtake them. In fact, some research shows that the harder you *try* to fall asleep, the longer it takes[4] – a phenomenon that you are almost certainly familiar with. Have you ever tried to get an early night because you know you are getting up early the next day, only to find that the pressure of trying to fall asleep inhibited sleep? Sleep is a homeostatic bodily function – meaning that your body tries to keep several functions in balance. One of these functions is sleep – the longer you spend awake, the more your brain tries to get you to slow down and, eventually, sleep will overtake you.[5] Your brain will literally slow down its activity, and despite your best efforts, you will succumb. Of course, you can resist sleep for a while – who *hasn't* ever stayed awake long past the hour they felt sleepy to finish a gripping book, cram for a forgotten exam, or stay up late talking with a new partner? You know you can do it! Willpower, coffee, determination – whatever it takes, it can be done. But babies don't think like that. They do sometimes get distracted and fight sleep, or get really unsettled, stressed or 'wired' and find sleep harder (more on that later), but eventually they will succumb, just like the rest of us. You do not ever need to teach them to do that. So, if you want to, you can forget all about sleep, and just carry your child around with you, knowing that at some point they will fall asleep.

What people usually mean is that children need to be taught to fall asleep with particular sets of cues, at particular times, or without parental intervention. That's another thing altogether. That's related to convenience and lifestyle-matching, not a normal bodily function. Like all of us, babies and children learn about what to expect through life experience. If they are repeatedly exposed to 'Twinkle, twinkle little star' from birth every time they shut their eyes, it is probable that over time, that song will be become linked to the experience of falling asleep. There's nothing wrong with that. There isn't even anything wrong with trying to get your child to nap *before* the school run, because you know that if they nap *during* the school run your bedtime will go belly-up. That's real life. However, there is a danger in believing that you need to teach your child to sleep in a highly prescriptive way. That's probably going to set both you and your child up for failure and disappointment.

Truth #4: Children have limited abilities to self-soothe

This deserves a bit of an explanation. First of all, we need to know what we mean by self-soothing. Do we mean the ability of a child to fall asleep with no support from an adult? Or do we mean the ability to calm down from a state of distress? There is a big difference. Often people mix up the definitions and the action, which is not helpful.

Back in the 1960s and 1970s, Thomas Anders was studying infant sleep. He noticed that all babies wake several times per night. No surprises there! But some babies were able to utilise some primitive skills, such as finger-sucking, and return to sleep without any parental assistance, provided of course that they weren't actually uncomfortable or hungry. Other babies woke in the night and needed help to go back to sleep again. The babies in the first group were dubbed the 'self-soothers' and the babies in the second group were referred to as the 'signalers'. The phrase was officially coined![6]

Another way of thinking about settling is when a baby or child is content and calm, and has just the right amount of tiredness, sometimes they can fall asleep unaided. This is amazing! This is also *not* self-soothing. In this scenario, the baby was already soothed and calm and simply fell asleep, which as we know from Truth #3, is a normal bodily function. Nothing magic happened.

If a baby or young child is crying, upset, stressed or dysregulated in any way, they will probably not be able to become calm without adult help. The reason for this is that the part of your brain that controls this ability is very under-developed at birth, and in fact goes on developing through adulthood. That's why even adolescents lose control and sometimes need help to calm down! It's just neurological immaturity. So expecting a baby to possess the advanced logical reasoning, problem-solving and self-awareness skills that calming down requires is ludicrous. Some babies have been shown to develop some limited self-regulating abilities from about the age of four months,[7] but these are very primitive – such as turning their head away from a scary stimulus, or thumb-sucking. But I must stress that not all babies seem able to do this, it may be related to temperament,[8] and even those that can will only have the ability to calm down from relatively minor upsets. Adults truly 'self-soothe' – they can get themselves from a state of stress to a state of calm by using a range of strategies or higher-order thinking skills.

So why do people say that babies will 'learn to self-soothe' if they are left to cry? Well, the reason I think they say this is because they have mixed up the two meanings that I have explained – the ability to fall asleep without help, and the ability to calm down alone. The two are completely separate. The child left to cry will eventually stop crying, and probably fall asleep, but it does not mean that any higher-order thinking occurred in their brain.

The other thing that parents often say to me is that their child *used* to be able to self-soothe and now they can't, or they have 'lost' the ability to self-soothe. The truth is that usually, children do not lose skills – in fact, it is a worrying developmental red flag if they do. So what has happened? Let's take the scenario of the child who peacefully falls asleep without help, and then for one reason or another ends up needing a lot of parental help to fall asleep. What happened is that before, either by accident or design, you got the moment just right – your child was calm and sleepy, and sleep overtook them. Now, their needs have changed, and they require something else to get them calm again. They didn't lose the ability to self-soothe – *they never had it in the first place*. It may be that your little one is going through a developmental change, their sleep needs have changed, they are more distracted, or whatever. But one thing is for sure, it is totally normal for them to need you.

Truth #5: You are not responsible for making your child fall asleep

You have many parenting responsibilities. That's pretty obvious really – you need to provide your child with food, shelter, safety, and love. You might at times feel like it is your responsibility to make your child sleep as well. This is not strictly true. You are required to provide a safe place for your child to sleep, and arguably it is also your job to get to know your child and provide the right environment, time or condition that will be conducive to sleep. But you cannot take responsibility for whether your child actually sleeps or not.

" I urge you to take the pressure off yourself and let go of the assumption or expectation that your baby will fit into your routine or achieve a particular sleep 'milestone'. "

It often feels like there is a lot of pressure on you, the parent, to get your child into a good sleeping routine, to achieve a certain number of hours of sleep in the day, the right number of naps, or have them asleep by a particular time in the evening. This is made worse by people whose babies do these things with seemingly no effort, but I assure you some babies are just like this. The truth is that you cannot force anybody of any age to fall asleep. I urge you to take the pressure off yourself and let go of the assumption or expectation that your baby will fit into your routine or achieve a particular sleep 'milestone'.

There's nothing wrong with wanting a more convenient sleep situation, and there are lots of gentle ways to make that happen, but I do think it's important not to take on too much responsibility for your child's sleep.

Truth #6: Your child's sleep is only a problem if it is a problem for you

That's right. As long as what you're doing is safe, you can carry on doing it. In fact, I invest quite a lot of time supporting parents to continue doing what they enjoy doing and ignore the negative comments from those around them. Other times, it's simply not the right moment to address your child's sleep. You may not have the energy, motivation or support to make changes. That's also okay. Don't be pressurised into doing anything you don't want to do. You and your child are not broken, and do not need fixing.

What makes one parent perceive a particular situation as problematic when another parent would perceive it as normal, or even desirable? Well, there are probably hundreds of reasons for these differences in perception. Sleep researchers agree that perception of sleep problems is greatly influenced by culture and the prevailing social customs that a parent is exposed to.[9-12] We cannot assume that everyone has the same tolerance for sleep fragmentation. But equally, we shouldn't assume that everyone will find the same scenario problematic either.

Truth #7: The way your child sleeps is not 'your fault'

Guilt comes up over and over again in conversations about parenting and sleep. Many parents believe that they are to blame for their child's current sleep situation, or that they need to accept that they have caused their child to sleep badly, or have been selfish in choosing to parent in a particular way.

It has been my experience over the years that most parents do the things they do to get their child to sleep because they have tried other strategies first. So, the strategy you now use is a *response* to the way your child needs to fall asleep, not the *cause* of it. For example, you might have already tried putting your baby down 'drowsy but awake', only to find that it didn't work. You then tried to pat and shush them, but they cried louder. You eventually ended up holding them in your arms because that was the only way they would fall asleep – you didn't rush straight to that. Even if you did – it's the most natural parenting instinct in the world, and it wasn't wrong. Even when you actually hate your current sleep situation, it still doesn't make it wrong. If you made a decision that was right for you and your baby at the time, it was the right decision. Period. In fact, this is pretty much the essence of responsive parenting – recognising and acting on the need that your child has, promptly and with compassion. In fact, some research has shown that being more emotionally available is linked with better infant sleep, possibly because the infant has a greater degree of trust in their caregiver and environment.[13,14]

Truth #8: Your child's sleep will improve

Honestly. Without you doing anything. You can make a positive choice to not do *anything*. You can carry on doing what you're doing and trust that at some point, when your child is ready, they will sleep longer, more continuously, and more independently. You may hear that poor sleep in infancy is linked with later poor sleep in adulthood. It's not true! Numerous studies have found that there is no correlation between broken infant sleep and later sleep problems.[15-18]

" This is pretty much the essence of responsive parenting - recognising and acting on the need that your child has, promptly and with compassion. "

Some babies seem to sleep through the night from an early age,[19] but there is considerable variability.[20] While some studies show that addressing infant sleep will reduce the number of night awakenings, other studies disagree, finding that the improvements are just temporary, and often need repeating, or that the reduction in night waking is not actually significant. So the jury seems to be out. I tend to support parents in a pragmatic and individual way based on what they tell me. If you are enjoying your current sleep situation but feel guilty about it, what you need is reassurance, encouragement and validation. If you're really struggling but lack the capacity to do too much about it, what you need is additional support, and some easy things that might help. If you're at desperation point, what you need are some sleep strategies that balance your need for sleep with your child's need for responsiveness.

I can promise you that all phases come to an end, and (nearly) all children eventually sleep well without intervention. Please do not address your child's sleep unless it really is becoming problematic for you.

Truth #9: Parenting is hard

You don't need me to tell you this. You already know it. They say it takes a village to raise a baby, and I'm sure that's true. In many countries, parenting really is a community activity, because many cultures correctly recognise that parenting in isolation is far from ideal.[21] Parenting in isolation can cause feelings of loneliness, low mood and poor sense of self-efficacy - that feeling of 'hey, I'm doing a pretty good job'.[22,23]

In countries where it is standard practice to remain at home and receive care from other members of the family, greater parenting confidence is reported,[24] and even in countries like China where this custom appears to be waning in popularity, in part due to Western influences, less postnatal depression and more parenting confidence are found among new families receiving social support.[25] It comes back to the idea from Truth #2 of valuing the role of parenting, and the acknowledgement that raising children is simultaneously profound, rewarding and exhausting.

I remember having a lightbulb moment during a mundane event that happens numerous times every day, up and down the country – mealtime. I remember serving my children their evening meal, feeling exhausted and, if I'm honest, a little starved of adult conversation and company. I heard our upstairs neighbours through the wall, as well as those to our right. They were serving dinner as well. My neighbour three doors down, and the one opposite, were undoubtedly doing the same. I had this crazy urge to knock on everyone's doors, close the road to traffic, put long trestle tables down the street and do kiddy dinner time *en masse*. How insane it suddenly felt to me that we were all struggling on alone, bored or lonely, and how the situation might be entirely turned on its head, to the benefit of children and adults alike, if we all had some company.

While it may not be practical or possible to enlist lots of family or social support to help you in the early days, weeks, or months, I'd like to encourage you firstly to accept help if it is offered, and secondly to find a village – even if your village is online. Very often, I meet parents who are trying hard to cope alone, fearing that accepting or asking for help will be viewed as weakness or incompetence. But in reality, recognising that you need help is one of the most sensible and self-aware things you can do. You are not weak to recognise your need for support – you're strong. Finding a 'tribe' of parents with whom you can be emotionally authentic and vulnerable, and who will support you in your parenting philosophy and decisions, is also really important. Because if you have plenty of social support in theory, but the 'support' isn't supportive, then this can actually have the opposite effect. That's why virtual support groups can be so valuable. You can spend too much time on social media, that's for sure, but if you find your village online, rather than in person, this is a good thing.

Truth #10: You are important too

You matter. I could leave it there really, because this is the truth. I don't particularly like the phrase 'happy mum equals happy baby'. I think it's a bit pithy, over-simplistic and belittles a lot of effort that some parents put in to do the best they possibly can. But I know where the phrase is coming from, and it's partly right. You, as your child's parent or carer, are their rock of security, and if you are calm, confident, content (most of the time!) and connected, then your child will almost certainly have a good outcome. But as I've mentioned already, parenting is a two-way street. You don't just want to feel this way for your child's benefit, but also for your own! How you feel matters. How you are coping matters. How you are sleeping matters. In our (very appropriate) efforts to be responsive, baby-centred and attachment-focused, we do not want to neglect our own needs. If you are holding your family together, but neglect your own needs, interests, and priorities, then parenting stops being a relationship, and becomes a job.

Sometimes we all need to hear a few home truths, especially in a world full of opinion, fake news and pseudo-science. Knowing the truth can validate what we do, put reason behind our instincts and confirm our belief in what we are doing. Surround yourself with truth, especially if those around you are trying to sway you from doing what you feel is in your family's best interest.

Chapter three

Optimising parent sleep

Why on earth is there a whole chapter on adult sleep in a book about infant sleep? It's a fair question. I'm actually a big fan of supporting adults with their sleep. Your sleep is important, but I have another motive too – it's easier. This is not about dodging the problem at hand or being lazy. It actually makes a lot of sense to do the easy things first. It is far easier to work on your own sleep, change your own habits, or modify your own behaviour, than it is to modify a baby or child's behaviour. If you can improve your own sleep, not only will this give you some good ideas for what might work with your child, but it also models good sleep habits to your children, and makes you feel better. If you are getting more sleep, the chances are you'll have more reserves, and a greater ability to cope with your child's sleep than you did before.

When I trained as a nurse, the big buzzword was 'family-centred care'. In practice, this meant that I spent just as much time caring about parents and siblings as I did my little patients. I made sure that the parents were comfortable, I made beds for them to sleep in, found them spare clothes when their child vomited all over them, or encouraged them to eat. I'm afraid old habits die hard, and I just can't let go of that ethos of caring about everyone. I truly believe that families only make sense in context, looking at every member of the family and considering everyone's needs. With sleep, it's just as true. If you only look at your child's sleep, you miss an opportunity to improve your family as a unit.

I'm not suggesting that you ignore your child's sleep altogether, but I certainly wouldn't make it the first thing you work on. You can review your situation once you've got your own sleep as good as you can get it. If your tolerance has increased thanks to the changes you have made, then you can leave your child alone. Even if you still find your child's sleep tough, you'll feel better having improved your own. You have nothing to lose!

What affects how you sleep?

To optimise your own sleep, you need to know about some of the factors that can influence sleep quality and quantity. If you know what affects your sleep, you can understand what you can improve, what you probably have to learn to live with, and which aspects are made more difficult when you become a parent. Sleep is usually best addressed in the context of lifestyle and wellbeing, rather than compartmentalising it.

Genetics

Genetics seems like a good place to start. Research studies disagree on the exact amount of influence that your genes have on your sleep habits, but all studies agree that this is a factor.[1-4] On a simplistic level, if your parents slept poorly, or struggled with insomnia, there is a chance that you will too. Of course, this goes for your children as well – which may be a depressing piece of news if you happen to know that you don't sleep well! Scientists are discovering new and fascinating ways in which our genes play a part in the way we sleep, how much we sleep, and our sleep patterns. You have genes that provide the code for whether you prefer to get up and go to bed late or early, genes that can be inherited for insomnia, and genes that make certain sleep disorders more likely.

In addition to this information about genetic influences on sleep, there is some new and exciting research that is revealing that our genetic code is not fixed, but affected by toxins, our environment, our relationships and nutrition. This is called *epigenetics* – the study of how information above your DNA can change the way genes are expressed. Basically, gene expression can be dialed up or down – rather like a dimmer switch. If you think about it, this is a good thing, because it allows us to adapt to our environment. Some epigenetic changes are really helpful – for example, the tendency towards being allergic can be dialed down by epigenetics. But it can also be unhelpful – for example, the tendency towards insomnia can be dialed up.[5-9] We don't want that! We are only just beginning to understand what factors may be responsible for some of these epigenetic changes. The research is still in its early days, but it seems that having a healthy lifestyle, and avoiding too much stress, are some promising areas to focus on.

Circadian rhythm

The other big influence on the quality and quantity of your sleep is whether you tend to get up and go to bed late, or early. This is known as your chronotype, and we all have a tendency towards preferring mornings ('larks') or evenings ('owls'). More recent research has suggested that there are actually sub-types of these preferences, and that there are 'bears' and 'dolphins' as well.[10] Bears seem to prefer to be aware during light hours – pretty much a 9–5 sort of preference. Bears apparently make up the vast majority of the population. Then we have dolphins – these sleepers make up only 10% of the population, but have a tendency towards light sleep, insomnia, and easily fragmented sleep. You will probably know instinctively which type you broadly fit into. Of course, it changes with age – you don't meet many 'owl' toddlers who enjoy sleeping in until 9am, and you will meet a disproportionately low number of 'lark' adolescents who prefer to get up at 6am and then have an early night.[11]

Your preference for being a lark, bear, owl or dolphin is controlled by a part of your brain known colloquially as your master body clock – it's official name is the suprachiasmatic nucleus, but I wouldn't worry about that! Your master body clock controls many other bodily functions that are related to the time of day. The reason that it can be so hard to cope with disobeying your internal body clock is that your body makes and releases hormones according to your unique biological rhythm.[12] If your master body clock is telling you that it is time to wake up, a whole cascade of physiological changes occur that are hard-wired to all your other body clocks around your organs and even at a cellular level. For example, you make more urine in the daytime, and then this slows down overnight (so you can get some sleep). If you always eat breakfast at 7am, pretty soon your appetite becomes linked to your body clock. You feel more alert soon after waking up, and begin feeling sleepy about 1-2 hours before your bedtime, under the influence of a clever little hormone called melatonin, which is released when light levels start falling. You only have to think about how disruptive the clock change for daylight saving is, to realise the profound effect your body clock has on your daily activity and functioning.

You can of course influence your chronotype to some extent, but the more extreme a chronotype you have, the less malleable it seems to be. Some people find that if they are an owl, they find it easier to get up early in the summer, because they are exposed to more daylight.[13] However, if you hate mornings and always have, the chances are that although you can develop strategies to cope, you will always prefer to sleep late if you have the chance.

Mental health

Your mental health also influences how you sleep, and the quality and quantity of your sleep. This can get pretty confusing, as mental health can affect how well you sleep,[14,15] but how you sleep can affect your mental health.[16] It's a classic chicken-and-egg situation. If you struggled with your mental health before you became pregnant and had children, then sleep deprivation may have made it harder for you to cope,[17] but it was clearly not the cause of your mental health problem. Whereas if you did not previously have a mental health problem, and then struggle with extreme sleep deprivation for two years, this may cause low mood independently. However, it's still not all that clear cut – after all, is a mental health problem caused just by sleep deprivation, or is it a toxic combination of social isolation, difficult adjustment to parenthood, and missing your old lifestyle? We need to be careful not to oversimplify human conditions which are very often multi-factorial.

Broadly speaking, depression and anxiety (which are the most common mental health problems to be studied from a sleep perspective) affect sleep in a few key ways. Firstly, someone who suffers with anxiety or depression tends to find it harder to fall asleep in the first place.[18] It normally takes about 15-20 minutes to fall asleep. If, for example, it takes 45 minutes to fall asleep, and not only initially at the start of the night, but also every time you are woken, you are losing a significant amount of sleep every single day. Secondly, a person with anxiety or depression also achieves less deep sleep – meaning that even after a 'full night's sleep' you can wake up feeling unrefreshed and fatigued.

Anxiety about your child's sleep can be particularly frustrating because as I have said, it is harder to change someone else's behaviour than your own. Feeling powerless and trapped regarding your child's sleep can be anxiety-provoking. It is common for parents to feel anxious about when and whether their baby will sleep, or whether they will feel this fatigued *forever*. One of the ways you can stay in control of anxiety is to understand that anxiety is often future-oriented. 'Will I ever get eight hours sleep?', 'What if my baby's sleep gets even worse?', 'What will I do when I go back to work?', 'How can I survive another six months on this little sleep?'. All of these anxieties are oriented in the future. They haven't happened yet, and honestly, they may never happen. The fear of something unknown or unquantifiable is often worse than the reality we live in. You can disarm the power of this type of anxiety by staying in the present. If you catch yourself thinking these future-oriented troublesome thoughts, remind yourself of what life is like right now. Even if your sleep is pretty dire, you're here. You're reading this book. You're taking action. Don't let anxiety dictate your next move.

Nutrition

If you thought nutrition was just about your weight and nutrients, think again. It turns out that nutrition may influence your sleep more than you think. The good news is that this is quite an easy fix – and who *doesn't* love a quick win? Broadly, nutrition can affect your sleep in a couple of key ways. Firstly, certain foods are either stimulating or soporific, and secondly, some nutrients are essential for the normal functioning of cells that are related to sleep.[19] Nutrients that are important for sleep include iron, selenium, magnesium, vitamins B12, C and D, calcium, potassium and zinc. At insufficient levels, these micronutrients are responsible for various sleep-related problems including non-restorative sleep (vitamin C, calcium), insomnia (magnesium, iron, vitamin B12), daytime fatigue (vitamin D, potassium, iron), short sleep duration and quality (zinc) and also certain parasomnias – such as restless leg syndrome and night sweats.

It would be nice if we could recommend a 'sleep-friendly' diet and that was all we needed to do. It's usually more complicated than this, but it is a pretty harmless thing to try. Just make sure that your expectations are realistic. Eating certain foods is unlikely to solve all your sleep problems, but it's a risk-free suggestion. Foods that may potentially help with sleep usually contain tryptophan, which your body uses to make melatonin (your sleep hormone). Try foods like turkey, bananas, spinach, almonds, cherries and lettuce. I challenge you to create a recipe that incorporates all those foods in one single meal! Turkey and spinach risotto with cherry and almond tart anyone? While we're on the subject, there are also some foods that may be stimulating, and therefore best avoided if you're struggling with sleep. For the best possible night's sleep, avoid high-fat foods which play havoc with your digestion, causing excess acid to be produced, as well as tomatoes and aubergines which both contain tyramine – a stimulant. Caffeinated drinks as well as chocolate are also not conducive to restful sleep – bad news for coffee and chocolate lovers.

The other nutritional aspect to consider is that if you are actually deficient in a nutrient that plays a role in sleep, circadian rhythm, muscle relaxation or the quality of your sleep, then this can be remedied by correcting the nutritional deficit. It's important to say that most people in the Western world are not deficient in nutrients, but an over-reliance on processed foods can make certain nutrient deficiencies more likely – especially magnesium, potassium and vitamin C. Vegetarians may find it harder to get enough zinc and vitamin B12. Nearly all of us are deficient in vitamin D. In general, if you eat a diet that includes plenty of fresh fruit and vegetables, and whole unprocessed foods and grains, you are unlikely to struggle. The problem when we are busy with young families is that it can seem like Mission Impossible to eat well. I vividly remember not really managing to cook a balanced meal for several months, and relying heavily on quick-cook foods like toast, cookies and the occasional apple – not exactly a diet to be proud of. If this is your predicament too, then please know that this is not meant to sound judgemental! I totally get it. But I wish someone had suggested to me that I treat food like medicine for my soul and my sleep. It might not have solved all my difficulties, but it might have helped me feel less sluggish and more energised.

Health and lifestyle

Finally, exercise, health and lifestyle can play a huge role in improving your sleep and stress levels. Getting plenty of exercise, nature time, and prioritising self-care can be game-changing for many people struggling with the vicious circle of fatigue, low energy and poor sleep. When you haven't slept well, it can be a real struggle to even contemplate getting your heartrate going! I can totally relate. However, I've been inspired to treat exercise like therapy. Start small – just have a short walk outside. You don't have to get all sweaty in the gym. It is also really difficult on a practical level to get a decent amount of exercise with small children in tow – so you may need to get creative. Hide and seek in the park? Get a baby seat fitted to the back of your bicycle? Dance around the house with your kids? There are lots of ways to be active without needing to find a babysitter or use the crèche at the gym.

Getting some exercise not only gives your body clock the right messages about what time of day it is, but will also give you a rush of endorphins and serotonin, which makes you feel better and boosts your mood. If we feel tired, the temptation to sit in the dark at home is strong. I call it 'cave mentality' – it's almost like we are trying to hibernate. But if you do this, your body gets a bit of a confusing message. You don't get exposed to bright light, so you may start feeling sleepy, but your internal body clock is trying to tell you that it isn't time for bed yet either. Although it can feel like the last thing you want to do, going outside in natural daylight is the best thing you can do, as it will wake your body up naturally.

How your sleep tolerance is affected by having children

However you slept before you became pregnant or had your children, you will probably have developed some habits, or coping mechanisms. If you struggled with your sleep, no doubt you managed to cope by using some hacks such as getting an early night, sleeping late the next day, or taking a nap. You only had to factor in your own needs, and if you have a partner, presumably, because they are an independent adult in a relationship with you, they would have given you the space and opportunity to do whatever you needed to do (within reason!). If it was necessary, you may even have been prescribed sleeping medication. You could go to an after-work Pilates class, or make time to meditate when it suited you.

Fast forward to children arriving on the scene, and many of these workarounds are not an option. That's not something you necessarily resent – after all, you love your children and understand that right now, they need you and that is more important than your early night. However, that doesn't mean it is easy! Adaptations after children are important to think about, because you may have been coping with borderline adequate sleep thanks to your ability to be flexible. Children are fabulous, but your average 18-month-old can't fend for themselves while you sleep late in the morning to compensate for the fragmented night's sleep you had, and nor would we expect or even want them to.

What I'm trying to say is that some of the effects on your sleep will be logistical and practical. The way you coped before may not be achievable or sustainable after children. You may need to rethink how you cope with reduced or fragmented sleep. You may also find that if your sleep was poor before you had children, your tolerance for night-waking is reduced because you don't have much of a buffer to protect you from sleep loss. You may therefore start to struggle earlier than someone who slept well before children.

How to help yourself sleep better

It is likely that one or more of these sections has jumped out at you – after all, nobody's sleep is perfect. You may find yourself feeling drawn to improve one specific area, or you might feel that multiple sections apply to you. In many ways, the more things that jump out at you, the more excited you can get. If there are many areas to improve, the chances are that you will see a real and visible improvement in your sleep once you start to address some of the variables.

There are some simple things you can do to help yourself, whether you are already a parent, or expecting a baby. These can be divided into three main areas:

1. **Relational improvements**
2. **Lifestyle changes**
3. **Sleep hygiene**

Relational improvements

This might seem a strange place to start, but if you think about it, having a stressful relationship is likely to negatively impact the quality of your sleep. Investing in your relationship, having someone around who can be emotionally available for you, and addressing problems within your relationship is likely to reduce stress and improve sleep.[20,21] Nobody has a perfect relationship, and there is always something you can do to improve the ones you have. Having children and becoming parents tends to have a massive effect on relationships – whether the one you have with your parents, your partner, your friends or siblings.

Becoming a parent may force you to reconcile the feelings you have about your parents and childhood. You may have had a wonderful childhood, or it may have been difficult. One thing is for sure, your parents (just like you) weren't perfect. There will be things that you won't want to repeat, and others that you want to become firm traditions. But add into the mix your partner's feelings, wishes and history, and this can make for some interesting discussions. We naturally lean towards the role models we had in our own upbringing – who may or may not be our parents – so if you and your partner had very different experiences, then you'll need to work out how to weave them into your parenting in a way that is respectful to both of you.[22] Perhaps try writing down – independently of each other – some happy memories, your parenting role models and anything that you feel is important to carry on. Use this as a basis for discussion.

Arguably the most significant impact is likely to be felt in your relationship with your partner if you have one. A renegotiation of time spent, activities, and role in the home is likely. This is exciting, but it is also stressful, potentially frustrating and can involve addressing issues that have never previously been tackled. If you are struggling in your relationship, please consider getting some help with it. Welcoming children into your life can bring a couple closer together, but it can also put your relationship under pressure. It is easy for resentment, comparison or criticism to creep in and chip away at the foundations you have with your partner. If you don't have the resources or time to see a relationship counsellor, then please consider talking to each other, a mutual friend, or someone who has known you both well for a long time. Being honest about how things have changed, and the good and bad aspects of those changes, can be a good place to start.

You will also have to work out the changing roles in the home. If you both worked before, but since having children someone stays at home – how does this change the allocation of household tasks? Previously you may have shared out tasks. If raising children is a full-time relationship/job, then who will do the household tasks? It is very easy for this to become the responsibility of the person at home, due to a perception that everything that takes place in the home is the job of one person. But is this realistic or achievable? Does this lead to burn-out or resentment? Is it possible to prioritise raising little humans with patience and compassion if the home environment is full of dirty dishes and laundry? These decisions are not easy to make or even the same for every family – they are worthy of open discussion.[23]

Lifestyle changes

Sleep is just one area of your health and wellbeing, but nothing really exists in isolation. Multiple lifestyle factors are interrelated, including health, nutrition, exercise and sleep.[24] For example, not getting enough sleep tends to affect what foods we crave, and the foods we crave might actually be stimulating and negatively affect sleep. Feeling fatigued might push us away from getting some exercise, but exercise is likely to help us achieve better quality sleep.[25] Eating well, and at regular times, has been shown to improve sleep and support circadian rhythmicity,[26] and in addition, eating certain foods, such as foods high in omega-3, might support sleep and lower inflammation.[27] These are just a few examples to illustrate why I believe that addressing sleep holistically leads to greater overall improvements and lifestyle satisfaction.

If you are struggling with your health – either physical or mental health – then please make yourself a priority. You are important, and you deserve to feel as good as you possibly can. If you struggle with your mobility, pain, stress, or function, then all areas of your wellbeing are likely to be affected. Please see whoever you need to see, get the referrals you need, and the treatment you require to make yourself feel well again. Raising children is a physically, emotionally, and psychologically demanding activity, and you will find it so much easier if you are in as good a place as you can be. If you have a chronic health problem, then please don't forget to come up with some new workarounds after you have children. The life hacks you used before might not be possible, but discuss with your healthcare team, family, friends and partner how you can manage your condition while also parenting and coping with sleep fragmentation.

Also decide today that you will treat food, exercise, and stress management like medicine. Make your own health and lifestyle a model for how you want your children to treat their bodies and health. This does not have to be overwhelmingly difficult. I recommend making one small change. Perhaps just go for a 10-minute walk every day with your child in a baby carrier or pushchair. Start a journal, use essential oils,[28,29] get a yoga for kids DVD and try it out with them, try mindfulness. Throw out food you know makes you feel worse, and decide that today you will have one extra portion of fruit or vegetables. I'm not talking about going straight from ready-meals to cooking quinoa and avocado salad (though that's awesome if you want to try it!) – just make some small changes and keep working on it.

Sleep hygiene

Improving your sleep hygiene can lead to overall improvement in the quality and quantity of your sleep,[30] and you can do this in many ways. Sleep hygiene is related to the habits and behaviours you have around bedtime, and the associations you make with your bed, bedroom, and bedtime routine. Developing an association between the bedroom environment and pre-bedtime ritual and a prompt and efficient process of falling asleep is the key to avoiding and managing insomnia. This sounds really obvious, but it is amazing how many improvements most people can make to their sleep hygiene. Here are some questions to ask yourself and consider:

- Do you go to bed and get up at the same time every day, including at the weekend?
- Is the bedroom only used for sleep and intimacy, with no screens, work, or big discussions taking place?
- Do you drink caffeinated drinks or alcohol in the hour or two before bedtime?
- Do you have a bedtime routine?
- Do you have a 'night' filter on any screens you use late in the evening?
- Do you set yourself boundaries about screen use in the evening and especially, do you enforce a 'no screens in bed' rule?
- Do you take naps in the day if you're tired?
- Do you exercise, but avoid strenuous exercise late at night?
- Is your bedroom pitch black?
- Is your bedroom a comfortable temperature?
- Do you set a time limit of about 20 minutes for falling asleep, and go to another room after this time if you're not asleep?

If the answer to any of these questions is no, then this is an area to improve. Full disclosure – even I can't answer 'yes' to all of them! I would encourage you to try to tackle the easy areas first, and be patient – it may take a few days or even weeks before the benefits of working on sleep hygiene are seen.

It is worth mentioning insomnia here. If you have ever had a night when you just cannot sleep, you'll be able to relate to this. Imagine that you have decided that you are going to get an early night. You get into your bed and lie down. You lie awake, with your eyes shut, trying to go to sleep. You may or may not have thoughts in your mind. You begin getting frustrated that your early night has turned into a normal night. Then a normal night turns into a late night. You begin to torture yourself by counting how many hours of sleep you will achieve if you fall asleep right now. Most people have had this experience at least once, but some unfortunately battle insomnia chronically. If this happens once or twice, there may be nothing you do except to write that night off as a disaster and move on. But if it happens a lot, then I urge you to get some specialist sleep support from your doctor. There are many strategies that can be tried, so if you've held off because you don't want to take sleeping tablets, don't worry – there are other options as well.

To treat insomnia, you have to understand it, and there are many different types and levels of severity of insomnia – so this is merely a simple explanation of sleep-onset insomnia.[31] Essentially, if you associate going into your bedroom and lying down in bed with a prolonged period of wakefulness, frustration and stress, then this is extremely unhelpful for sleep hygiene. You need your bedroom, feeling sleepy, the bed and the process of falling asleep to be associated in your mind with going to sleep promptly. You will want to address the easy things as well – such as screens, caffeine, stress. You can also expose yourself to light in the daytime and a variety of other environmental cues such as noise, social activity, eating and interaction[32] to regulate your body clock. You could also try a technique called bedtime fading. If you battle insomnia, one approach that has been found to be highly effective is cognitive behavioural therapy for insomnia (CBTi). It encompasses various strategies such as sleep restriction, challenging unhelpful or negative beliefs about sleep, and relaxation.[33] Sleep restriction warrants some explanation – as it sounds rather counter-intuitive to the average tired reader! Essentially, you would delay your bedtime until the latest time that you have fallen asleep over the last week. So *regardless* of when you went to bed, what matters is when you fell asleep. Keep track of this for a week (some phones or watches are able to measure when you go to sleep). Then do not allow yourself to even get ready for bed until 10 minutes before this time. If necessary, even getting ready for bed in another room can help. The aim is to link the action of going to bed with rapid sleep onset – to correct the negative sleep association. Once you are falling asleep quickly (within 15-20 minutes) you can begin to gradually shift bedtime earlier, but maintain all the positive sleep hygiene habits you have established. There are, of course, other techniques and strategies, so please do not suffer in silence if this is a significant problem for you and simple strategies have not helped. While these simple self-care and sleep hygiene ideas may work for many, it is important that you see your doctor if simple solutions do not work for you, or you have other concerns about your sleep and wellbeing.

Catch up sleep?

Finally, it is worth mentioning naps. You have almost certainly had someone give you the advice to 'sleep when the baby sleeps'. It is not necessarily bad advice, but it is not always as simple as it sounds. I'd like to bust some myths and get realistic here. First of all, the baby has to *actually* sleep for that to be possible. They have to sleep for a long enough period of time for it to be worthwhile. They also have to sleep somewhere that does not require your intervention to maintain sleep – so if your baby only sleeps in the baby carrier, or your arms, or the pushchair while being walked (all of which is common and normal), then this advice is useless. The other problem is that sometimes, when there is pressure to fall asleep, it can be very hard to achieve a rapid onset of sleep. Some people are great at power-napping, while others find it extremely difficult. I have known many parents who lie awake, desperately wanting to nap, but subconsciously waiting for their baby to wake up. I've known others who enlist help for an afternoon so that they can catch up on sleep, only to get a burst of energy and end up doing housework or catching up on social media instead. The point is, this piece of advice is not wrong, but it might not be universally applicable.

Naps have indeed been shown to improve concentration, memory, performance, learning and ease the heavy feeling of sleepiness known as sleep inertia. They contribute to positive sleep hygiene and are definitely

> **Working on a fully verbal, logical adult's sleep is a hundred times easier than working on the sleep of a tiny human with immature thought processes and high needs.**

a good idea.[34] I was once training a group of maternity nurses and nannies, and at the lunch break, one nanny checked her watch and then announced that she was going to take a nap. She rolled up her sweater and used it as a pillow, draped her jacket over the table to create a darker space, and then lay down under the table. She set an alarm for 20 minutes and woke up refreshed, fully engaged for the rest of the afternoon. I was in awe – mostly because I wished I could do that – yet despite the number of times I have tried, that technique doesn't work for me. If you can do this, and you have the opportunity to power nap, then do it! Research suggests that power naps are extremely good for your concentration and productivity. A study measuring the effects of naps of either 10 or 30 minutes following a sleep-restricted night of less than five hours sleep showed promising improvements in functioning.[35] Another study acknowledged that although there are cultural variations in the prevalence of napping, many people use naps throughout their lives to cope with sleep deprivation, fatigue, shift work, or just because they enjoy it.[36]

Being pragmatic about napping, if you are able to nap, and have the opportunity to nap, then go for it. If you have the opportunity but would actually find something else more restorative – whether it is reading, Pilates or just lying down without the expectation of sleep – then do that instead. If you need to achieve something, like studying, answering work calls, or housework, then reframe this positively in your mind: you are doing something constructive and positive with your time. I remember feeling so frustrated by the state of my home that actually, the idea of lying down felt stressful. I found it therapeutic to tidy up so that my *environment* was less stressful. That's okay too. Do what relieves your stress levels most effectively – whether that involves slowing down or speeding up.

If, however, you would love to nap but cannot because your baby is not sleeping in a way that facilitates your nap desires, or your child has dropped their nap, then I want you to have some practical strategies too. Firstly, could you put your baby in a baby carrier and either get tasks done while your baby sleeps, or go for a walk? Sitting outside or getting the grocery shopping done while your baby naps might be a pragmatic option so that you don't have to negotiate the shops with a child who is awake later on. Could you adjust your expectations of rest? For example, if your baby is a short napper, or needs your presence to remain asleep, could you just rest on your bed and let go of any expectations to achieve anything? No social media, no emails, no typing 'how to get baby to nap better' into google, or anything else that might cause you stress. Simply lying down or resting on your bed can feel at the most luxuriously indulgent, and at the very least, a chance to put your feet up and slow down for a few minutes.

Hopefully it is now obvious why working on your own sleep is a good first step. Not only might your sleep not have been perfect before your children came along, but your coping strategies might also need to evolve. There are many quick-fix ideas that might give you modest improvements in your sleep without going anywhere near your child's sleep habits, and let's face it, working on a fully verbal, logical adult's sleep is a hundred times easier than working on the sleep of a tiny human with immature thought processes and high needs. By addressing the obvious areas for improvement in your sleep, it is likely that you'll feel better quickly, have a greater tolerance for the sleep fragmentation caused by your child, and you'll also be modelling positive sleep habits for your family to copy. You have nothing to lose. Even if you are still struggling after working on your own sleep, it will be a lot easier to make changes to your family's sleeping habits if you have addressed the basics first.

Chapter four

Positive sleep starts in pregnancy

→ This chapter is for you if you have ever been pregnant, currently are pregnant, know someone who has been or is pregnant, or work with people in pregnancy. Basically, everyone. Why? Because pregnancy induces some pretty profound changes to sleep and functioning. Understanding these changes can bring meaning to the symptoms you experience, or explain the behaviour of the loved one in your life. I am mindful as I write that not everyone becomes a parent in the same way. There are many wonderful routes to parenthood, including surrogacy, fertility treatment, and adoption. I'm also very conscious that not everyone who is pregnant identifies as 'female', 'mother', or 'woman'. It is not my intention to exclude anyone, so please know that I support, acknowledge and welcome all parents, regardless of gender identity, sexual orientation, or fertility status.

Pregnancy is a hugely dynamic and fascinating adaptation that necessitates changes to almost every single body system to accommodate a healthy growing baby.[1] People have varying ways of adapting to and

"Pregnancy is a normal human condition and is not a health problem." coping with the changes during pregnancy: some people report that they have never felt better, while others want to fast-forward the whole process. How people cope with pregnancy is therefore both highly individual and intensely personal. It is also a time when parents-to-be are sometimes bombarded with questions, advice and comments, both from the general public and also health professionals. It is almost as if carrying a baby gives people licence to offer up way more information than is strictly socially appropriate. Suddenly people want to share birth stories, tales of procedures and anecdotes about various examinations or interventions.

People also often love to offer unsolicited advice, or ask intensely personal questions about how you plan to care for your baby. This is where you can really start getting confused, and it is certainly the case with sleep. Let's face it – you have a lot of decisions to make. Things you didn't even know were 'things' before you knew you were expecting become something else to make a decision about. There are products for wrapping your baby, transporting your baby, changing your baby, feeding your baby, playing with your baby, and, of course, sleep products. All of these products are marketed in a way that promotes sales. I have to say – the vast majority of them are unnecessary. Some are hugely overpriced. Some are odd, and some are actually dangerous. It is of course your parental right to buy whatever you want and can afford for your baby. But please know that there is not a product available that will make your baby sleep. Save your money and invest in hiring a postnatal doula instead.

General changes that accompany pregnancy (and may cause fatigue)

If you can get past the unsolicited advice and booming baby product industry, there are many changes that take place in a pregnant body. Understanding them might help you develop a new-found respect for pregnancy. Knowing about these changes might also help you cut either yourself or the person in your life some slack.

Everyone's experience of pregnancy is unique, and despite the adaptations that occur, some people breeze through pregnancy with no or few complaints. Pregnancy is a normal human condition and is not a health problem. I mention these changes not to scare people or pathologise pregnancy, but merely to bring understanding to the fatigue that is commonly experienced. This is important, because there is a tendency to blame fatigue on a new baby, when actually many people are already experiencing fatigue and sleep changes *before* their baby arrives. In fact, according to one study fatigue seems to worsen at about three months post-birth,[2] so it may not be the newborn phase that causes fatigue.

Physical extra load on your body

No getting away from it. When growing a small human, your body needs to increase in size, weight, and metabolic rate.[3,4] This is no major surprise – after all, you're growing arms, legs, a digestive system and an entire new person. Your heart will work 20 percent harder, and your circulating blood volume will increase by 50 percent. Pretty incredible really. Despite the higher blood volume, the red blood cells do not increase in production at the same rate, which means that many women experience something called dilutional anaemia.[5] This is why most pregnant women have their blood tested to make sure that they have enough red blood cells. If not, they may be prescribed iron supplements to support them.

With all that increase in physical size and the subsequent shift in the centre of gravity, there are some physical changes that have been found to be associated with lower health-related quality of life – including back and pelvic pain.[6] Some women really struggle with aches and pains, while others, as I have said, really enjoy their pregnancy and don't find it uncomfortable.

Immune changes

There are many adaptations that your body will make to keep your unborn baby safe. Many people think of pregnancy as being an immune-suppressed state, but this is not strictly true. Rather, the immune system is modified, with some parts of the immune system protecting the unborn baby from being rejected by the maternal immune system, and other parts of the immune system being very responsive to bacteria which would pose a threat to the baby.[7,8] Pro-inflammatory cytokines rise in the third trimester to support the immune response, though these molecules are also implicated in depressive illness.[9,10] The complex immune function changes necessary to sustain and support an unborn baby may take 3-4 months to return to pre-pregnancy levels.[11] The stress-response mechanism is also altered in pregnancy, which leads to an increase in a molecule that regulates blood sugar and suppresses the immune system. It's pretty awesome really that your body is able to differentiate between pathological invaders, yet protect the foreign body that is your baby.

Mood, sex drive and body image

Ask anyone who has been pregnant about mood swings and you will get a volley of responses. Some people experience joy, contentment, or peace. Others find the changes in their body unsettling and uncomfortable, and they resent the changes to their physical appearance. There has actually been a lot of research exploring attitudes to body image during pregnancy over the last few years. As you might expect, people's responses to their body changes are varied, and may relate to the relationship they had with their body before they became pregnant. They may feel liberated or invaded, feminine, cumbersome or out of control.[12,13] There is no *wrong* way to feel, but there are certainly more *positive* ways to feel. Developing positive body image – or at the very least, making peace with your body – has been shown to improve psychological wellbeing, and is also important to factor in with breastfeeding decision, as shorter breastfeeding duration is associated with body image concerns.[14] Negative body image is also associated with depression, so it may be a warning sign to seek help with your general feelings about your body and mood.[15] One study found that developing an attitude of gratitude and mindfulness during pregnancy was associated with a more positive outlook on physical body changes and greater satisfaction – so this could be something to explore if you're struggling in this area.[16]

As well as body changes, and the associated feelings about this, pregnant women (as well as co-parents) might also experience changes in their sex drive.[17] Many people are cautious about sex initially, and towards the end of pregnancy, but the second trimester is highly variable across couples. It is likely that this is related to sexual activity before pregnancy – so if sexual dysfunction was present before pregnancy, it is likely to continue during and afterward too.[18] While most couples can anticipate that having children will necessitate some adaptations, it is important to find other ways of continuing to nurture and sustain relationships during reduced physical intimacy.[19]

Anxiety is another commonly reported symptom during pregnancy, which may have an impact on sleep and general functioning as well.[20]

Several studies[21-23] have found that anxiety and mood disorders are common in pregnancy, and may be similar to a grief response – which actually makes sense on a number of levels. Gaining a baby means a loss of independence and freedom. The transition to becoming a family also involves self-sacrifice and putting another's needs before your own. Of course, this is a wonderful and beautiful thing, but it is okay to feel a sense of loss of your former life as well – that doesn't make you a bad person! It is important to normalise anxiety and not make the anxiety itself something to feel anxious about. You may be anxious about yourself, your birth, your baby, parenting, or even sleep.

Many people experience anxious thoughts in their everyday life, and have found ways of managing it so that it doesn't become a barrier to their everyday functioning. I have met several people who have become anxious about being anxious. If this is something you can relate to, then I strongly suggest that you explore ways of managing your anxiety. Don't beat yourself up about feeling the way you feel, simply acknowledge it and try different strategies to help yourself. For some people that might be mindfulness; others like journaling. Some people use exercise as a way to manage their mental health, while others practise self-compassion, self-care and self-forgiveness. However it looks for you, know that you're not alone.

Nausea

Nausea and vomiting are common and were found in over 30% of pregnant women in a large study.[24] Fatigue as an independent symptom in early pregnancy was found to be a factor in over 40% of women in the same study. Nausea and vomiting are usually experienced in the first trimester, but some women suffer with them throughout their pregnancy, or have hyperemesis gravidarum.[25] Nausea can affect your appetite and eating patterns, so can have quite a profound effect on your quality of life and functioning. A recent study[26] found that nausea and vomiting during pregnancy required a careful balance of normalising, and not over-medicating, but without trivialising the problem and making women feel dismissed. For mild symptoms, ginger has repeatedly been found to help, as has eating small, bland, frequent meals, while muscle relaxation has also shown promise.[27] More severe symptoms do occasionally require medication or hospitalisation.[28]

Nighttime toilet trips

I can almost hear the groans of women as they relate to this. It is undeniably annoying to have to get up to go to the toilet in the night. Many women report that they are scared to drink too much in the evening because they know they will pay for it with nocturnal bathroom visits. Frequent urination and difficulty finding a comfortable position to sleep in were experienced by approximately 80 percent of a recent sample of pregnant women, with all women in the sample reporting night awakening during pregnancy.[29] There is almost nothing you can do about this, besides reassure yourself that it will pass (no pun intended). The only other possible remedy is to avoid drinking caffeinated drinks, especially in the evening. Caffeine is notorious for increased urine production, so experiment with non-caffeinated drinks and see if that helps. Otherwise, you have my sympathy!

What about partners?

If your partner is pregnant, you matter too. You are also affected by pregnancy. Not only are you witnessing the metamorphosis of your partner, dealing with weird food cravings and trying to be endlessly patient with mood swings, but the chances are you are also experiencing some mood changes, anxiety or stress as well as dealing with the change in your relationship. Pregnancy is an amazing time - nobody is denying it, but it is also hard on couples and a lot to get your head around. Your adaptation to pregnancy and the feelings you have around it will probably be closely linked to the quality of the relationship you had with your partner prior to becoming pregnant.[30] One study found that younger fathers were at greater risk of depression following the birth of their babies, and anxiety about finances was also a trigger for low mood.[31] Another study found that fathers felt left out, and would have appreciated more information about the transition to parenthood, breastfeeding, and the changing relationship with their partner.[32]

What about co-parents in same-sex relationships?

For people in same-sex relationships, there may be an additional narrative of feeling like you don't quite fit in.[33-35] Some lesbian co-mothers describe frustration, anger or distress at not feeling that their role is important or understood. In one study, the theme repeatedly arose that their needs are the same as everyone's but not completely.[36]

For parents expecting a child through surrogacy there are additional complications if a close relationship cannot be established with the surrogate prior to birth, with gay men in one study reporting feelings of frustration and disconnect due to geographical constraints.[37] A recurring theme is the need for social support from friends and family who are supportive.[38]

What about transgender co-parents?

Transgender parents may also encounter difficulty and opposition during pregnancy. Although increasingly the needs of people who do not identify with their birth gender are being addressed, there remain many barriers and social stigmas. I am genuinely in awe of the bravery of transmen who conceive, carry and give birth to their babies after socially or medically transitioning to their male identity. There are a number of research studies which have identified the need for non-discriminatory, individualised and compassionate care. There are also some identified specific areas of difficulty, including social isolation, accessing information that is targeted to 'women', and gender-stereotyped literature, as well as body dysphoria.[39] There are also important considerations and conversations that transmen need to have after birth – such as whether to chest/breastfeed, and whether supportive, knowledgeable care around the management of chest or breastfeeding is available. Please find an empathic breastfeeding counsellor or IBCLC who is familiar with supporting transparents to chest or breastfeed if you need further support.[40] You will probably also find considerable support within online communities specifically created for transgender people birthing and breast/chestfeeding – Facebook is a good place to look for allies.[41]

Pregnancy after a loss ('Rainbow pregnancy')

This section comes with a trigger warning – please do skip it if this is not what you need to read right now. First of all, if you have lost one or more pregnancies then I'm so sorry. There are lots of feelings to come to terms with during a 'rainbow' pregnancy. You may feel grateful, anxious, on edge, angry, sad, or a bewildering combination of all of those emotions and more. I do not attempt to know how you feel, even though I myself have lost several pregnancies. Everyone's experience is unique and meaningful. There are, however, some common themes that emerge from parents who have suffered a pregnancy loss. These include trauma, anxiety, sleep changes and depression. That doesn't mean that everyone who suffers a miscarriage, ectopic pregnancy or termination will experience any or all of those, but there seems to be an association.

Recent studies have found that those who experience pregnancy loss have lower general health, social functioning and mental health than those who have not suffered a loss.[42] This may mean that your ability to connect with other pregnant women is more strained because your experience of achieving a successful pregnancy is different. You may find yourself wondering how you can relate to someone who became pregnant 'easily', and seemingly had no problems.

Some research suggests that anxiety about the pregnancy loss is commonly experienced until about six months after the loss. This particular study highlighted the importance of reassuring parents that anxiety will usually diminish over time.[43] This is important, because so often we expect to be able to be happy all the time. The truth is that it is normal to feel sad after sad things happen. Allowing parents who have lost a pregnancy to feel sad and to acknowledge their anxiety, without over-pathologising it, is important to normalise the recovery process. The issue might be more acute if another pregnancy comes soon after the loss. Compassion, patience and understanding are always needed, but perhaps more so after a loss – and that's not just from your healthcare providers: be compassionate and understanding to yourself too.

Pregnancy loss is associated with trauma, depression and sleeping problems, especially if you suffered with anxiety or depression before you became pregnant.[44] Most studies find that having someone to talk to about the feelings experienced after a bereavement is helpful. Not all parents will want to receive counselling, but at a bare minimum, having someone available to listen openly can be very therapeutic.[45] The support available to women should be culturally appropriate and respectful. Another recent

"Grief that is not processed can develop into a 'debt' against the next pregnancy."

study explored the needs of young black women who had suffered a perinatal loss. These women needed culturally sensitive support, and valued physical mementos of the baby they had lost, such as footprints, as well as community and faith support.[46] I would urge anyone who has experienced a pregnancy loss, for any reason, and at any stage, to seek support if they are struggling. As one recent study so eloquently put it; 'Grief that is not processed can develop into a "debt" against the next pregnancy'.[47]

A pregnancy loss can also directly or indirectly affect your sleep – with one study reporting an association between losses and disruptive dreams in the next pregnancy. After a stressful event, your brain's attempt to process information can result in more REM sleep, leading to more dreams, and less restorative deep sleep, which can be a cause of fatigue and daytime sleepiness.[48]

Sleep-related adaptations

Some of the adaptations I have mentioned already will have an indirect effect on sleep. Not all of them are changes you will have noticed, and the same might be true of sleep adaptations. Towards the end of pregnancy – from 36 weeks onwards – nearly 80 percent of women in one study reported sleep difficulty[49] as well as insomnia, lack of energy and drowsiness. You will probably have at least one person tell you that sleep disturbance in pregnancy is 'good practice' for when you have a baby. I don't know about you, but I find that most people who have been told this get really annoyed by it. It does a few things. Firstly, it can instill fear. There is no need to fear sleep with your newborn. You already know it will be different, and your sleep will be interrupted. But you will also be waking up to care for a tiny human whom you love more than you could ever have imagined. It's not something that needs to frighten you. You'll be okay. Secondly, it dismisses the difficulty that you might be struggling with right now. If you're having a hard time, and you've been brave enough to share that, you don't need to be patronised and given a strange explanation for your loss of sleep. You need proper explanations and some practical tips. Thirdly, it's kind of irrelevant. Your baby isn't here while you are sleep-deprived in pregnancy, and you can't actually prepare for lack of sleep. Certainly, a lack of sleep before an event that will probably cause further sleep loss is not helpful. Manageable – yes. Normal – yes. But does it prepare you for your baby? – I think not. You'll have to smile and nod and learn to ignore comments like that I'm afraid.

It's amazing really how few areas of the body are untouched by pregnancy. You will experience changes at an organ, cellular and microscopic level. All the changes have a distinct purpose and do not happen by accident. One of the most specific sleep changes that occurs is the adaptation of the circadian rhythm. You might wonder why this needs to be affected by pregnancy. Your circadian rhythm affects much more than just when you wake up and when you go to sleep. It also regulates hormone production, cardiovascular function, repair of damaged tissues and temperature regulation. Certain immune responses are enhanced in the daytime. Your circadian rhythm also controls your sleep hormone, melatonin – which fascinatingly also has an important role in reproductive health and pregnancy. Melatonin is also made by the placenta, and is transferred to your unborn baby to give vital information about hormone metabolism and other important functions.[50] It is therefore unsurprising that on closer investigation, your circadian rhythm would be affected by pregnancy in a very profound way – it is a vital way of keeping your unborn baby safe, and managing the additional physical workload of the pregnancy. You actually have circadian clocks at organ and cellular level too, which control numerous functions from appetite to urine production, and immune activity to temperature.

Melatonin is a really important hormone of pregnancy, and more is produced by the placenta than in the brain. Melatonin is a powerful antioxidant and also has a crucial role in ingesting harmful bacteria, and may be important for the developmental programming of your unborn baby's immune system. Melatonin is also an anti-inflammatory and may have a role in preventing inflammatory mediated conditions such as preterm labour and pre-eclampsia.[51] And people thought it just made you sleepy!

During pregnancy, instead of one circadian rhythm there are essentially three: mother, baby and placenta. It appears that the changes to the circadian rhythm are important for coping with the high metabolic demands of the growing baby, and for managing the immunological challenges of not only keeping the baby safe from infection, but also not rejecting the baby as a foreign invader.[52] Circadian rhythm changes continue in the postpartum period, often made worse by lack of exposure to light. But these changes often start to become marked even before the birth of the baby, with sleep duration becoming shorter and more fragmented in later pregnancy.[53]

The expression of genes which control the circadian rhythm seems to be affected by estradiol and progesterone. What this means in practice is that the hormones released to maintain the pregnancy affect your body clock in a meaningful and observable way. Estradiol rises during pregnancy and dramatically falls after birth – which is hypothesised to cause more problems with insomnia, mood swings and temperature changes because estradiol is used by your body to make serotonin (one of your 'happy' hormones), and in turn serotonin is used to make melatonin. We've already seen how important melatonin is for regulating your circadian rhythm and helping you fall asleep. It's not a huge surprise therefore that if your body has a sudden dip in the chemical 'ingredients' it needs to make your sleepy hormone, that you might have difficulty falling asleep, and problems with temperature control.

How sleep may be affected

Hopefully by now you are both in awe of the human body, and totally unsurprised by the massive changes in energy levels and functioning during pregnancy. Almost every single body system is affected by growing a new little human, and it is therefore completely obvious that this should affect sleep, mood and energy levels. Your sleep may be affected in a number of ways – the quality, quantity and pattern of sleep. It is known that the general 'work' of pregnancy is associated with poor sleep quality[54] on quite a general level. Poor sleep quality is usually defined by a number of markers – such as how long it takes to fall asleep, the sleep duration, sleep disturbances, daytime sleepiness, and sleep efficiency – which is the amount of time you spend in bed versus the amount of time you are actually asleep.

Insomnia is a common complaint, as well as other parasomnias, such as sleep-disordered breathing and restless legs.[55-57] Restless legs are most common in the third trimester, and may be caused by or worsened by low iron levels. Restless leg syndrome causes uncontrollable urges to move the legs, often due to a strange tingling, aching or burning sensation that is relieved by movement. It can happen at any time, not just during pregnancy, is generally associated with low ferritin or iron, and usually improves after correction through increasing dietary intake of folate and iron, or through supplementation.

Sleep-disordered breathing, including sleep apnoea, mouth-breathing and snoring, is also more common in pregnancy. It is thought that women are more at risk because of weight gain and the shift in your diaphragm which is caused by your little one taking up space in your abdomen – which leaves less room for your lungs (which is also why breathlessness is a common symptom during pregnancy). Certain pregnancy hormones also seem to cause some narrowing of the upper airways, which may cause snoring. These symptoms are usually improved by sleeping on the side, and not the back.[58]

It is also important to end this section by acknowledging that it is not just *being* pregnant that causes tiredness. It seems just *living* with someone who is pregnant causes fatigue as well. A recent study found that fatigue and stress were common in both parents.[59] This is possibly for two reasons: firstly, all the toilet trips, snoring, and tossing and turning might wake up partners, and secondly, I wonder if some of the fatigue experienced by parents-to-be is caused by anticipation and anxiety about the impending arrival of their baby. Could it be that future parents are subconsciously mulling over those big questions – 'Will I be a good enough parent?', 'What will my baby be like?', 'How will our relationship change?' and 'Am I ready for this?'. It is normal and common to have fears and questions. This is a major life change and frankly, I'd be surprised if you didn't have some pretty big questions on your mind. Your life will indeed be changed in multiple ways. But you, like millions before you, will be okay.

What might help?

It is most supportive if sleep problems can be addressed during pregnancy, as some studies have shown that poor sleep in pregnancy is strongly associated with depressive symptoms after birth. This suggests that while it is common to blame fatigue and depression on infant sleep patterns, the problem may pre-date the birth of the baby.[60]

One of the first things that might be transformative is to rethink sleep, pregnancy and your body.

Body image

Rather than focus specifically on sleep, it may be helpful to develop some more positive ways of thinking about your body and baby, and their impact on sleep. I have met people, (and I have even been this person) who have indirectly blamed their pregnancy for how they feel. This is really understandable on one level, but it is probably not helpful. Developing a positive body image[61] can positively influence your mood and your sleep. I often encourage people to think about sleep in a roundabout way. So often, if you put pressure on yourself to go to sleep, it just won't happen. But if you concentrate on working on the things that are preventing you from feeling good about yourself, or relaxed, then this often has an indirect positive influence on sleep. So rather than think (as I did) 'I can't sleep because the baby is squashing all the air out of my lungs/bouncing on my bladder/won't stop wriggling', try to reframe it positively. For example, developing an attitude of gratitude might look like: 'Tonight I am grateful that I have a lively baby who is developing a personality', or 'Well, hello baby – thanks for reminding me that my bladder is working hard right now to keep you strong and healthy'. It is certainly a discipline, and might not come naturally, but over time you'll learn to develop a positive version of the things that are getting you down. Everyone has a different perspective regarding body image, physical adaptations, sex drive, stress and coping mechanisms.[62] Developing a new-found awe and respect for your body can help you to forge a bond with your baby.

Filter out other people's unhelpful remarks

I'm afraid I have no solution for unsolicited advice, comments or intensely personal questions. The truth is – some people will always do that. Maybe they don't realise what they're doing, or that what they are saying could be unhelpful. Maybe they do. Either way, unless you suddenly develop the ability to create a thick skin, you'll have to avoid conversations or people you find unhelpful, let it go over your head, or develop a comeback. Deflecting the comment on to the person who said it is an option. Or you could try the age-old smile-and-nod tactic. Or if you're feeling witty you could have a stockpile of responses you churn out at opportune moments.

A slightly more supportive suggestion is to remind yourself that mostly, people make comments or offer advice – no matter how unhelpful, misguided, or inaccurate – because they care. Allow that fact to be the prevailing one you take away, rather than the content of what they said. They probably mean well. More importantly, try to find yourself a tribe of like-minded people who are non-judgemental and with whom you can be real and raw.

Optimise your sleep as best you can

The next practical suggestion is to try to optimise your sleep as much as you can. This will involve some hacks to make the best of your current situation. You probably won't sleep seven or eight hours straight, so you will have to let go of that as an expectation. What you're trying to achieve is the best possible sleep for you and your body, in your current situation. That is all you can do. Don't feel bad about what isn't possible; instead, make some small changes and try to only work on what might be possible.

Firstly, don't fight your body. When we slow down and listen to our bodies – I mean *really* listen to them – it is amazing what they can tell us. If your body tells you to eat, then eat. If you feel a powerful urge to nap, then nap. If you do nap, set a timer for 30 minutes. There is pretty good evidence that a nap of longer than this can make you feel worse. You could feel groggy or disorientated, or not able to sleep at night if you nap too long. If you're still working, then allow yourself a 10-minute power nap during your lunch break. While we are on the subject – make sure you *have* your lunch break! It's amazing how often we forget the basics. Eat at regular intervals, try to avoid caffeine in the evening, drink plenty of fluid in the day but consider not drinking too much in the hour or two before bedtime. Set a time limit on screen use, have a soothing bedtime routine, and try to lie on your side.[63] These things sound so simple that sometimes we doubt whether they will be effective, but I assure you, simple is often the way to go.

Diet and exercise

If you struggle with shopping, cooking or eating then this may not be easy. Personally, I love to cook, but I get stuck for inspiration and end up making the same things over and over. Planning the family's meals is the most boring conversation of the week in our home! So, this is not intended to sound preachy. Eating a healthy diet – especially eating enough fibre and fruit and vegetables – will really help the way you feel and boost your energy levels. In fact, some research has shown that it helps your sleep as well – which makes sense, because if you have insufficient nutrients, or a condition that is exacerbated by poor diet, then eating well will self-correct this. A classic example is constipation, which is common in pregnancy, probably caused by progesterone which can slow down your gut motility. Drinking more, getting more exercise and eating plenty of high-fibre foods, including fruit and vegetables, will almost certainly help.[64] If you struggle with inspiration, motivation or the skill needed to cook and prepare healthy food, then I would urge you to focus on what the barriers are. Is it time? If so, could you cook ahead of time and freeze portions of food? Is it inspiration? Try a boxed weekly meal scheme to take the thought process out of planning meals. Is it nausea or the fact that you don't feel great? Is there a time of day when you feel better and could cook for later on? Is it tiredness and fatigue? If so, think of food as medicine. Everyone has a different lived experience of pregnancy symptoms and unique challenges, so trying to figure out what your particular issue is will help you to focus in on strategies that are achievable and most likely to make a difference.[65]

Exercise might feel like the last thing you want to do if you are feeling uncomfortable, nauseous, tired or all of the above. It may require a significant amount of willpower, but it is almost certain to make you feel better. The trick with exercise is to find something you like - you're more likely to stick with it. Low to moderate muscle-strengthening exercise reduces fatigue and boosts energy levels and maintains healthy weight gain.[66,67] Try swimming, walking or gentle resistance classes in a gym. If that's not your thing, then yoga has been shown to be safe, reduces stress and improves sleep.[68]

Practise self-care

It seems that as a nation we are getting better at talking about mental health and self-care. Being kind to yourself is really a very wise strategy. It can be too easy to think that we have to keep on going the way we did before, or to be just as functional as we were before we were expecting a child. It is ok for you to call these lies out. You *have* changed, and your life *is* changing. Embracing this and letting go of unrealistic expectations of yourself is a great idea.

One good place to start if you're not sure where to begin is with your morning routine. In his highly successful book, *The Miracle Morning*, Hal Elrod[69] suggests starting the day with six habits. First, start your day with silence - perhaps try just giving thanks for the day ahead or try a guided meditation or relaxation. Next, tell yourself some affirmations – starting your day with positive self-talk will help you to feel motivated, calm and less negative. Then visualise how your day will go. See yourself achieving your goals and think about what you need to get done today. After this, do some exercise – it could just be some yoga poses, or stretching, or walking the dog. Next up is to do some reading – it doesn't have to be much, maybe just read a part of a book that is inspirational, or try reading a biography of someone you greatly respect. Finally, scribe – write something down. It could be what you'd like to do today, or what your hopes for your baby are.

Having healthy, positive habits is one thing that many successful people agree on. If you find it hard to adopt a new habit, then many people recommend 'habit stacking'.[70] What this means is to 'stack' the new habit on to an already established habit. So if you have decided you will eat more fruit, eat the fruit at the same time as your established breakfast habit. Another way to get a new habit is to create a 'to-do' list and check off the habit once you've done it. It can take time for habits to become established, so starting something alongside your partner is another option. For example, if you have decided to get more exercise, why not exercise together so you can motivate and encourage each other? Starting a new habit is often relatively easy – we are fired up and motivated. Eventually, habits become hard-wired and we cannot imagine not doing them, but it's the time in between that is the hard part.

As you move through your day, allow yourself time to stop. You might need to rest, nap, change task, eat, do something that makes you feel better, or talk to someone. If you need help, then please can I urge you to ask for it. Whether you ask a friend, colleague, family member, your partner, or a health professional, it is not a sign of weakness to ask for support. In fact, it's good practice. After your baby arrives you will need help, and what's more, people are likely to offer. Get into the habit of saying 'Yes please' rather than 'Don't worry, I'll be okay'. Getting help is a smart move – even CEOs delegate tasks!

Finally, develop a positive attitude towards sleep. Sleep is not a battleground. You will find that developing positive habits around sleep, and developing a positive dialogue about the sleep changes you are experiencing, will reduce the stress you might feel. Doing something constructive can have a remarkable effect on your outlook, and starting with small, achievable goals is less likely to set you up to fail.

Can you expect your sleep to be the same during pregnancy and early parenthood as it was before? Absolutely not, but you can have healthy and realistic expectations. Starting these expectations in pregnancy will hopefully mean that you continue with your modified view of 'normal' sleep once your little one is here.

Chapter five

Relationships and sleep

→ You might wonder why this chapter is here. What does your relationship have to do with sleep? Well, it probably doesn't take much thought to realise how much your relationship might be affected by sleep deprivation. But is it possible that the quality of your relationship might have an effect on sleep? Well, it turns out that it does. Poor relationship quality or stress is associated with poor quality sleep among adults, as well as children.[1] Poor quality sleep is associated with more arguments, sniping and tension.[2-4]

It is difficult to measure normal sleep deprivation effects on parents and their social functioning, as there are so many variables. Studies can be extreme. In one study, significant sleep deprivation (56 hours of wakefulness) led to some specific symptoms – all of which are highly relevant to relationship functioning. These included depression, anxiety, paranoia, self-doubt, hostility, perception of unfairness, blaming others, and sensitivity to perceived criticism and mistrust of others.[5] Importantly, these symptoms were within normal ranges and did not mean a formal diagnosis of a mental health condition. This study was also testing some pretty extreme sleep debt, which we need to bear in mind. But, if you can recall a time when you have been extremely sleep-deprived, I'm sure you can relate to feeling distinctly different on a psychological level than when you are well-rested. It is not surprising that after a couple of really disturbed nights many parents can therefore feel that they are becoming depressed, when in actual fact they are just severely sleep-deprived.

When one parent is getting more sleep than the other

Does the primary carer role always become synonymous with the person who sleeps less? How do gender roles affect the allocation of tasks? In your family do you actively embrace, reluctantly accept or actively reject gendered roles within parenting, and how does this change if and when both parents are working?[6] Gender roles are also complicated by financial decisions, areas of strength, and personal priorities. For example, will the parent who earns more return to work because it makes more financial sense? If this is the case, how is the 'workload' of the parent who stays at home quantified in a meaningful way so that they feel appreciated, valued and recognised for their household contribution? How do parents make decisions about childcare when one parent desires more strongly than the other to stay at home and care for their child? None of these are necessarily easy conversations or decisions. If you have this all worked out then I totally salute you, but in case you struggle with these topics, here are a few areas for further thought or discussion. Working out what the underlying emotion is could be the key to improving the relationship you have with your partner. Is there a recurring theme? Do you tend to have the same fight but after a different trigger every time? Ask yourself how you are actually feeling. This is by no means an exhaustive list.

Recognising negative emotions

Guilt is a weapons-grade self-esteem damaging emotion. Do you feel guilty for going to work and leaving your partner at home when things are tough? Do you feel guilty for not being patient 100 percent of the time? Do you feel guilty for staying at home while your partner gets up and commutes into work? Sometimes incidents or situations arise where we really could have handled a situation better. We might lose patience, snap, or react badly. This is all pretty normal, but the way you respond to these events may have a significant impact on your feelings of self-worth. Choosing self-compassion is a much more constructive response to incidents that could otherwise induce guilt, blame and shame,[7] but this may be something that needs to be prompted. This is where another partner can be hugely helpful to channel their co-parent towards self-compassion, rather than shame and guilt. For this to work, it is obviously better if you're both on board with this strategy and return the favour when needed.

Resentment can also sneak into a relationship. Resentment occurs when there is an underlying injustice (real or perceived), or a sense of being made to feel small or insignificant.[8] You might resent your partner for getting a full night's sleep – especially if they then declare that they are tired! You might resent your partner because they are able to spend the day with adults, go to the bathroom without an entourage, or manage to drink a hot cup of coffee. Or you might resent your partner because they get to spend all day at home. You might imagine that your partner spends their day in luxurious relaxation, not fully aware of the minutiae of events that occur during the day that are stressful, difficult, or just plain annoying. Frustration, anger and disgust often accompany resentment – so this is a pretty noxious combination of feelings that needs to be recognised and addressed. If it is, because it is often brought about by a sense of being unfairly treated or made to feel inferior, addressing those triggers can spark behaviour change, improve relationships and lead to a cessation of these unpleasant feelings.

Jealousy is fairly similar to resentment, but there are subtle differences relating to wishing you have something that someone else has. It might come from just one of you, or you may harbour feelings of jealousy – for example, your partner may be jealous that you got a full night's sleep, while you may be jealous that they get more time with your little one. It may be related to the primary role you have. 'I miss going out to work', or 'I miss our kids when I'm out at work'. Jealousy can be managed by validating the feelings you have about a situation, learning to accept it, and practising mindfulness and self-care.[9]

Imbalance is another emotion to potentially contend with, and may mean imbalance of power, imbalance of respect/value/appreciation, or

> **" We don't always need or want a problem to be 'fixed' – sometimes we all need to just offload. "**

imbalance of workload. If you feel there is an imbalance, take some time to check what you mean. If it is to do with something practical, such as workload, then specifically what is it that you're finding difficult? There are three main areas of workload for most couples: paid employment, household chores such as cooking, cleaning and laundry, and caring for children. How these roles get allocated can be the root cause of a feeling of imbalance. If it is more of an imbalance of power, value or respect, then work out what is driving that feeling. Is it an absence of gratitude? Making a specific and practical suggestion about how you would like your partner to treat you in order to feel respected and valued is a good idea – they may simply not have realised.

Competition is extremely common, especially when it comes to fatigue: 'We're both tired, but I'm *more* tired' comes up a lot. The root of this is often feeling like your efforts are unnoticed or invisible. Sometimes, the person staying at home feels the need to justify the fact that they are not in paid employment by stating how much harder their new role is, or how much more tired they are. This is probably symptomatic of our culture that does not value the importance of parenting. If it was universally acknowledged that parenting children was a vital role, both on an individual and familial level and also on a community and societal level, then perhaps we wouldn't feel the need to justify how 'busy' we are. It can also be related to feeling unappreciated or taken for granted. Finally, it can also be a cry for help. Perhaps one parent declares how exhausted they are, and counts the hours of sleep that they have had, in an effort (consciously or subconsciously) to validate their need for a break. The other parent may also be tired, but tries to explain why they are tired, despite getting more hours of sleep, because they don't feel they have the capacity to help out any more. If this happens, it is a burnout situation, and you may need to rope in extra help, or think practically about how you can work as a team to help both of you get more rest.

Moving towards positive emotions

Obviously, we'd all rather deal with positive emotions! I expect there are a few here that you can relate to. Try to recognise them and build on them if you're already doing something really well. If you struggle to see any of these, then consider how you could start to build some of them into your relationship.

Understanding is a good place to start. This doesn't necessarily mean everything will be wonderful, but starting with hearing where your partner is coming from and acknowledging what they are saying is really supportive in itself.

Empathy is defined as the ability to understand and share the feelings of others. Being empathic is probably the most constructive thing you can do, and the good news is, there are some really easy ways to demonstrate empathy. You've probably heard of the phrase 'walk a mile in someone else's shoes' – this is exactly what empathy is. It is the ability to truly imagine what another person must be thinking and feeling. It requires the listener to withhold judgement and personal bias and instead choose to put themselves in the position of their partner. Empathy can be really hard when competitive parenting has sneaked in – one parent may feel like their partner doesn't 'deserve' their empathy because they are 'less tired', or 'less overloaded', or whatever. So although this sounds simple, it is often a conscious choice to be empathic. You may even need to choose to be the 'bigger person' and be kind first. Once you have got your head around this, a few useful questions include: 'Will you tell me how you're feeling?', 'What is it like to be a parent from your perspective?', 'It sounds like neither of us have had a great day – do you want to share?', 'I'm really sorry today has been so hard. Is there anything I can do to help?'. I can pretty much guarantee that you will not make the situation worse by asking these questions and thereby letting your partner know that you not only understand what they have told you, but you are also trying to understand how they feel as well.

Compassion is empathy moved to action. Compassion is a practical emotion that drives people towards solutions. For example, you might hear that your partner has had a terrible day, and you can really imagine how difficult it must have been for them. You are moved to try to do something to help. What you do will obviously depend entirely on what the problem is. So, if your partner says they are feeling exhausted, compassion might move you to offer to take the children out early so that they can go back to sleep.

Redistribution of other roles to lighten the burden is a practical way of addressing overload and burnout. We don't always need or want a problem to be 'fixed' – sometimes we all need to just offload or complain about something and receive some sympathy. Other times, we really need practical help. It doesn't have to be permanent, but it can really help in an emergency when one person is struggling.

Respect and appreciation are also positive ways to try to feel about your partner. There is almost always something that can be valued or admired in someone else. Respect comes from a profound sense of honouring someone for who they are, what they do and how they do it. Does your partner go to work uncomplainingly? Does your partner get up in the night with grace and without sighing? Do they always have a smile for your little one regardless of how many curtain calls there were after bedtime? Acknowledging the tasks, character attributes and hardships that your partner has and manages to do is enormously uplifting. Sometimes our 'work' – wherever that takes place, can feel invisible. Acknowledging it basically says 'I see you. I saw what you did, and I really appreciate you for that'.

When one parent is significantly struggling

At some point, one parent may become extremely tired and if the other parent is willing, this may be a time to step up the hands-on nighttime support. This can 'rescue' a situation that is getting out of hand and allow some sleep recovery in order to continue.

There may be many ways of dealing with this, which we will revisit in the chapter on sleep crises, but a few quick ideas include:

- Getting home earlier from work to be more available at bedtime.
- Leaving late for work so that your partner can get some catch-up sleep to compensate for their disturbed night.
- Working from home.
- Taking some annual leave/vacation to be more present and available.
- Dividing the night into 'shifts' and allowing your partner to get some solid hours of sleep while you take care of your child until it is your 'turn' to sleep.
- Alternate nights so that you both have a chance to sleep.
- If you choose to bed-share, is there a way of making this even better?

Helping your partner out before they reach breaking point is a really compassionate thing to do, and may prevent both of you choosing a more hardcore strategy that you later regret. I spend a lot of time working with people who are desperately tired, but have sought help while they still have the motivation to choose a gentle strategy to improve sleep. The danger of waiting until a crisis is that the situation may become so urgent that you feel pressure to address sleep more decisively. So, supporting each other and making sure that you can prop each other up is a family-centred strategy that captures the fact that every member of the family affects every other member of the family. You need to think of the family as a whole unit: if someone is having a hard time, it will eventually affect all of you.

When parents have different perspectives on sleep management

This is where things can get a little awkward. It's actually pretty unusual to find a couple who are entirely on the same page with almost all areas of their parenting, childcare philosophy, discipline and sleep management. If you are – this is awesome. But for those of you who are on different pages, I imagine that this causes some interesting discussions from time to time. Often one parent has more of a lean towards gentle strategies, and the other leans towards stricter, or tough-love strategies. This may not just relate to sleep, but may transcend other areas of parenting and discipline.

I don't necessarily have an easy answer to this problem. In an ideal world, parents would either be on the same page, or they would have this discussion before a child arrives. But in reality it's not always easy to predict which issues you need to deal with. You don't always know in advance which areas you might potentially disagree about. Sometimes we assume certain things about our partner based on previous situations or discussion, and only when a new problem comes up do we realise there is a difference in opinion, priority or philosophy.

When it comes to agreeing how you will parent, you may need to work this out as issues arise. Take an online parenting course, attend a class together, or read a book on parenting. Make time to discuss the specifics with your partner afterwards. I would suggest that with sleep, rather than fall out about exactly how you manage the sleep situation, ask each other what you like about the current situation and are unwilling to change, what you'd consider changing, and what you definitely want to change. The possible outcomes are:

- You want a change and your partner wants the same change
- You want a change and your partner will consider a change
- You want a change and your partner will not consider changing

Obviously the same is true the other way around, and in reverse, but you get the idea. The most difficult situation is one where you want opposite things. Everything else can be negotiated. But wanting opposite changes is hard. For example, your partner wants to bed-share and you are vehemently opposed. Or your partner wants the children to go to bed later so they can see them when they get back from work, and you want them in bed earlier because otherwise they are cranky. You will have to each give your points of view, and see if there's a compromise that you can make.

How is your relationship with your baby affected by sleep changes?

Becoming a parent changes everything. It changes your outlook, your role, how you spend your time. That means that if you are struggling with parenting for whatever reason, it can affect your self-esteem – after all, if you are struggling with the role you spend a lot of time, effort and love on, you can begin to feel inadequate. It is why you will have to learn to trust that the measure of how great a parent you are is not how easy you find it, nor does it depend on objective and measurable outcomes like how 'well' your little one feeds and sleeps. You are a great parent if you love unconditionally and put your child's needs first. Whether you find parenting easy, enjoyable, difficult or frustrating does not affect how good a parent you are. If you are finding it tough, this is a sign that you need more support, not that you are getting it all wrong.

Many children are hugely longed for. There might be heartache, waiting, medical treatments, investigations or loss along the way. When the long-awaited pregnancy arrives, sometimes parents feel like they should be grateful, uncomplaining or always happy. I've met many parents who felt that after waiting for a child for several years, they felt guilty for complaining about pregnancy sickness, or aches and pains. They had to embrace *everything*. Even the parts that most people complain about. When sleepless nights come, they 'can't complain', because *at least they have a child*. Your mind can play some vicious tricks on you. There are two truths here:

1. You might have signed up for parenting, but that doesn't mean that every moment is total bliss. You are allowed to find some parts difficult or even annoying. You signed up for sleepless nights, but you don't have to love that. That's okay. That doesn't mean you don't adore your child. If you have a bad day and question yourself endlessly, you just need more support. Or a hug. Or a hot bath. Or anything that makes you feel like you are a normal parent who is struggling with normal parenting.

2. Just because you want to complain about parenting and sleep sometimes, doesn't mean you are asking for a solution. This doesn't mean you *have* to find a solution. It's okay to just want to complain and have nobody offer a strategy or solution to 'fix' it. If you find that people offer solutions when you just want to offload, I recommend two things. Either, offload where nobody can offer advice – such as in a journal. Or preface your complaint with 'Just so you know, I just need to offload – I'm not asking for solutions...'

Your relationship with your child can easily become bound up with how you are finding the transition to parenthood. Revisit chapter two and remind yourself that you are enough for your child. If this is you, then I want to encourage you to separate the challenges and your perception of your parenting role from how much you love your child.

This might seem almost taboo, but I'm going to say it, just in case you feel like this and nobody has ever said it out loud: it is not that unusual in your most sleep-deprived and frustrated moments to blame your baby for how exhausted you feel. That doesn't mean that you don't love your baby. It doesn't mean that you need to read anything deep into your feeling – sleep deprivation can make us irrational.[10] I've said it before, but I'll say it again – you might have signed up for sleep deprivation, but it doesn't mean you have to like it. If your partner wandered in to the house after you'd gone to sleep and woke you up you would probably (unless you happen to be a saint) be pretty annoyed with them and blame them the next day for your broken night's sleep. Babies wake their parents up in the night, and for the most part, parents attend to them selflessly and patiently. But personally, I would be lying if I told you I'd never groaned out loud at being woken up again in the night. I would be lying if I told you I'd never looked at my children when they were babies and thought:

'Gosh I love you, but oh my goodness I wish you hadn't kept me awake all night' (or words to that effect). Again, feeling this way does not make you a bad person or a bad parent. It also doesn't necessarily mean you want solutions. Having a chance to offload and complain to someone might be all you need. If so, find someone who will allow you to do what you have to do to feel unburdened.

The impact of co-parenting on infant sleep and parental stress

Co-parenting is the term used to describe two parents (of any gender) jointly parenting a child or children. What is the relationship between working together to raise children and sleep quality? Well, as you might imagine, like many other areas, this tends to go in both directions. That is to say that working well as a team tends to positively influence sleep, and poor sleep tends to affect the perceived quality of the co-parenting relationship.[11] So, as well as working gently on everyone's sleep – starting first of all with your own sleep – you could come at this from another angle and consider how the relationship you have with your partner could be improved in order to improve sleep indirectly. Although it seems hard to believe, having a strong relationship, that is high on praise, warmth, cooperation, and respect, independently improves infant sleep even if you do nothing else. Whereas a relationship where there is lots of criticism, complaints, belittling, and patronising is associated with poorer sleep. Sometimes, the specific challenges that parents face as a team can actually forge closer links, in spite of their reported struggles with sleep deprivation, such as when parents are caring for a child with autism, for example.[12] Developing ways to stay close despite the challenges, whatever they are, will reduce stress, improve cohesion and improve sleep.

There are many reasons why relationships may be under pressure. The change in dynamic, adaptations of role, and adjusting to have another person in the relationship can all be tough. Throw sleep deprivation into the mix and the situation can become highly charged. And this assumes the relationship was starting from a solid base in the first place. If you were struggling before children arrived, those issues probably haven't gone away, they've just been buried under more current and urgent issues. I don't pretend to know your unique situation, so I can't offer specific support, but there are many areas that you and your partner could consider in order to improve your relationship, reduce stress, increase your own sleep and improve your child's sleep.

First of all, you could decide to allow equal priorities of work and family life. Without both work and family life functioning well, neither can flourish as they need to. Think of your roles as equal but different, but I would strongly urge you to think of housework, cooking and laundry as joint responsibilities. It may be more practical for one person to *do* a particular job, but that doesn't make it their *responsibility*. This is about allocation of resources. Too often, if 'childcare' and housework get lumped together, what happens is that the person with these dual responsibilities feels overworked. Caring for children is a full-time responsibility, and the housework, cooking and laundry is another full-time responsibility. The only sensible thing to do is to divide this. That doesn't mean that the jobs need to stay static – take this on a week-by-week basis. If your partner has an end-of-year bulge in workload and needs to put in extra hours, then that might mean a reallocation of jobs. If a child is sick and one parent has been up all night, then despite it being technically that parent's job to take the bins out, cut them some slack. Strengthening parenting alliance improves parenting self-efficacy and reduces stress.[13]

Secondly, you could choose to listen with empathy to the other parent's point of view. Seeing the situation from another person's point of view is a good starting place with this. It takes huge willpower if you're feeling angry or resentful, but force yourself to listen actively. Take turns to say exactly how you feel, and the other parent should listen without interrupting, correcting, disagreeing or putting their own viewpoint across. Then summarise what your partner just said. Here's the kicker – you summarise even the points you disagree with! Ouch. This takes discipline. Some simple ground rules that can be helpful include:

- Don't try this in the heat of the moment. Wait until you're both calm, then initiate a discussion.
- Decide that you will use 'I feel' statements, rather than 'You make me/ you do this' statements.
- Avoid using the words 'never' or 'always' – they instantly get people's backs up. People tend to immediately think of the exception to the statement, rather than focus on the sentiment behind it, which is often feeling taken for granted, overworked, or underappreciated.
- Take turns to talk.
- Decide to listen without judgement. This is very hard, as you will

instinctively want to defend yourself, or act as the judge and jury, but this won't get you anywhere.

- Acknowledge that the objective is not to decide who is 'right' and who is 'wrong', or who has been 'wronged', but to find a solution to the problem.
- Try to see the problem as outside of yourself. I often talk about imagining that the problem is in a box. You and your partner sit down at a table, and place the problem on the table to talk about it without attaching fault or blame to each other. The *problem* is the problem, not your partner.

This might sound like: 'Okay, you told me that you feel irritated because from your perspective you do bedtime most evenings'. Don't forget, feelings are always valid. They are not always accurate, but they *are* valid. You might have an internal inventory of the times you've done bedtime and feel personally attacked by this perspective, but allow your partner to say how they feel. So, the response, when it's the other parent's turn, might be: 'I feel frustrated that when I get home, you're already in the middle of bath time, and I don't want to come in at that point and start getting the kids all excited. So I try to stay out of the way. I miss you and the kids, but I'm trying to help, and then I feel like I get blamed for not helping in the right way.' Allowing someone to tell their side of the story, using the ground rules, means you might get somewhere. When you take the blame and finger-pointing out of the situation, you often uncover the underlying hurts, misunderstandings or different perspectives. It's simple, but extremely effective at allowing other people to feel heard and validated. Once it's all out in the open, then you can begin trying to find solutions.

Thirdly, you might want to think about how you could redefine 'teamwork'. We've already been through the decision to allocate equal prestige and responsibility to caring for children and working for money. When both roles are treated with respect, partners usually feel more supported and less unappreciated. I would suggest that you make this a daily negotiation. Caring for children shouldn't be thought of as a 'job', and yet there are many tasks that need to be done: running the bath, making the evening meal, cleaning up after the meal, picking up dirty clothes – you get the idea. Some people are naturally more intuitive about anticipating the jobs that need to be done – and this can mean they end up doing them all by default, because it is quicker than explaining to someone else when or how to do it. But if this happens, resentment can creep in, and one person risks burnout. If you are the naturally more intuitive one, consider laying out the 'tasks' and allocating them jointly. For example: 'Okay, tonight can you clean up and load the dishwasher, while I go get the kids in the bath?', or 'Do you want to do bathtime or stories tonight?'. Constant negotiating without assuming that one person will always take on the same responsibility avoids one parent feeling stuck. Cooperation and involvement is a good way to reduce stress and overwork, and has been shown to improve infant sleep.[14,15]

Fourthly, ban criticism. Criticism can be one of the most damaging weapons in a relationship. Frequently being told that we are not meeting someone's standard can lead to low self-esteem and defensiveness and can break down intimacy and trust. It can easily slip in to conversation, especially during flash points or times when everyone is tired, stressed or there are many tasks that need to be done. For example, 'You've done the nappy up too tight', 'She doesn't like being held like that', 'You're doing that wrong, give it here', or 'Why did you only read one story – I always read two'. If you think about it, the natural response would be 'You do it then!'. If you feel like your efforts are wasted, not good enough or invisible, then the natural response is to choose self-preservation and retreat.

Finally, consider being flexible in your approach and strategy. What works for everyone else might not work for your family. It's totally fine to think outside the box. Maybe tag-teaming at bedtime works for you. Maybe you alternate roles. Perhaps you do something completely different on work-from-home days.

How to keep a healthy distance between sleep and relationships

Separating tiredness as a direct result of sleep fragmentation and short sleep duration, from fatigue that results from the overwhelming responsibility of becoming a parent is a good idea. We often blame tiredness on sleep disturbance, but I cannot tell you how many parents I've supported who tell me that even after sleep has improved, they are still tired. It's like a dawning realisation that their fatigue was not all about sleep disturbance. Adjustment to the new role of parenting can be mentally draining. Being *needed* can be exhausting, and feeling 'touched out' can be overwhelming. But these feelings are not necessarily just about sleep. Acknowledging the other factors implicated in your tiredness levels can help to keep a normal perspective, and maintain realistic expectations about yourself, your child, and family life in general.

It is also a good idea to make time to discuss practical household matters, as well as for distinct quality time, as this has been shown to reduce stress and improve the quality of relationships.[16] If there isn't protected time to deal with household 'admin' and parenting issues that crop up, then these vital conversations can spill over into time that you set aside to just hang out and regroup as a couple. Work out when you can catch up on the 'business of the day' and then your time to relax – even if that is just 10 minutes while you snatch a hurried meal – is time just for you as a couple. It's so important for household admin, child-related dramas and bills not to crowd out your time together. If you're stuck for conversation, I recommend investing in some Table Topics cards. These are conversation starters with intriguing and thought-provoking questions – a lifesaver when you can't think of anything intelligent to say!

Redefining parenting as a relationship, not a job, shift, or burden is exceptionally important. Changing language can help. Instead of 'I've got to take the kids to school', say 'I get to take the kids to school', or instead of 'I've given up my job to take care of our children', try 'I'm able to stop working corporately to care for our children'. These subtle language shifts, when woven into the narrative of our day, can redefine caring for children as a positive and privileged role, rather than a burden.

Developing coping strategies can also help. In one study of working parents, practising mindfulness improved work-life balance.[17] Mindfulness and working on specific areas within the couple relationship may help to get to the bottom of the underlying cause of stress, which is also likely to improve sleep.[18]

The bottom line is that having children changes every relationship you have. Learning how to embrace the changes, make space for new people, and adjusting expectations can make you better people. Although parenting could be the most challenging role you have ever had, it also has the potential to make you into someone you never thought you could be. A humbler, gentler and funnier version of yourself – if you allow it to.

Chapter six

Normal infant and child sleep

→ Most children have no diagnosable sleep pathology, but the paradox is that almost all parents struggle with their child's sleep at some point. In many cultures we have come to think that if something is really hard, then there must be a problem. In lots of ways, this is an appealing idea, because if there is a problem, there is often a solution. To be told something is 'normal', can therefore come as a disappointment, because that means you either need to persevere, or try to change something that is actually normal – which as you can probably guess, is not easy. However, if you can get your head around normal sleep, you will realise that there are probably some easy things you can do to improve sleep without doing anything you feel uncomfortable with. Let's start by understanding infant and child sleep.

Circadian rhythm and homeostatic sleep pressure

Stick with me – this is actually quite important, and nowhere near as boring as it sounds! Your circadian rhythm is your body's biological clock,

> **" Your daily circadian rhythm is controlled by your body clock, which organises your sleep-wake cycle with a combination of hormones, environmental cues and differences in body function. "**

and affects your sleep-wake cycle, certain bodily functions and activity levels. Your body clock continues to tick along, irrespective of whether you are awake or asleep – that's why you feel out of kilter when you have jet lag. Your body clock has carried on ticking, and it takes a while to adjust.

In the womb, an unborn baby is exposed to the maternal circadian rhythm. The baby receives cues about the time of day from their parent's activity levels and environmental cues, as well as maternal production of melatonin and cortisol, which the baby is exposed to via the placenta. As we learned in chapter four, the placenta actually makes melatonin as well, because it appears that melatonin is a vital hormone for many functions as well as sleep.

Melatonin is the hormone which increases the drive to fall asleep, and it is released in response to dim light.[1] It mainly affects nighttime sleep, as levels are virtually undetectable in the day. Melatonin is a circadian-linked hormone and levels are higher at night, falling in the early hours of the morning and remaining low during the day *even while daytime naps occur.* Melatonin is therefore not the only reason you fall asleep, otherwise you would not be able to fall asleep in the daytime. Melatonin doesn't work like a sleeping tablet, or sedative – it just makes you feel sleepier, and in the mood to go to bed. Melatonin begins to be secreted in most infants from about one month of age, but does not reach stable levels until about three months.[2]

Cortisol has a bit of a reputation as the 'stress hormone' and indeed it *is* released at times of stress. You have to remember that we need to be able to respond to stress as humans. Otherwise, if there was an imminent danger or threat, we would be too chilled out to respond promptly! A healthy stress response is a lifesaver. But an unhealthy stress response is an entirely different matter – we'll cover this more in the next chapter. Cortisol, for the purposes of sleep, is also released on a cyclical basis, with higher levels in the morning, and the lowest levels about 3-5 hours after nighttime sleep onset. Cortisol levels rise on a month-by-month basis over the first 12 months,[3] but then fall between the ages of 1-6 years.[4] Cortisol helps you to feel alert, so it makes total sense that you would want more of this in the morning as you start your day, and less when you're trying to fall asleep. Cortisol has many other functions as well, such as maintaining your blood sugar, and it is also an anti-inflammatory – but these functions are less relevant for sleep.

There are other circadian fluctuations that are unrelated to cortisol and melatonin. For example, there are variations in your blood pressure, and urine production – so you don't need to use the bathroom as much at night. Your appetite is also circadian-linked – so you feel hungry predictably first thing in the morning, and at regular times in the day, but you do not wake up at night feeling hungry. If you go on holiday and have to deal with jet lag, one of the most annoying things is that you feel genuinely hungry at strange times, because your internal body clock has not yet caught up with the local time zone. This change in appetite is linked to differences in activity level. Basically, in the daytime your metabolic rate is higher and you are burning more energy because you are active. At night, in the resting state, your metabolic rate is reduced, so you have a reduced need for calories.[5] Infants and children have higher metabolic rates and are undergoing phenomenal amounts of brain development, especially under the age of two, which may explain why they continue to be genuinely hungry at night.

Your body temperature is also circadian-linked. It is highest in the evening, and lowest in the early hours of the morning. Funnily enough, sleep seems to be highly influenced by core body temperature. This makes a lot of sense if you think about your personal experience. How many times have you tossed and turned, unable to fall asleep because you are too hot? Or woken at 3am freezing cold? In fact, a drop in body temperature seems to trigger sleep, which is why you can't fall asleep if you're too hot. Melatonin seems to be responsible for the drop in body temperature, though there is much less evidence that taking steps to lower your body temperature will increase melatonin production. In other words, melatonin affects temperature, not the other way around.[6]

So, your daily circadian rhythm is controlled by your body clock, which organises your sleep-wake cycle with a combination of hormones, environmental cues and differences in body function. All of these develop at different rates. If we imagine a sleep developmental timeline from birth, it would look a bit like this:[7]

One month: Immature cortisol and melatonin rhythm starts. Core body temperature rhythm emerges.

Two months: Differences in sleep state emerge. More sleep achieved in the night than the day.

Three months: Response to light and activity levels are circadian-linked. Melatonin reaches stable levels.

Six months: Circadian rhythm is generally mature.

As you can see, this is not a quick process. Often, I hear from both parents and professionals that the expectation is that sleep will consolidate around three months, because many people are aware of the fact that melatonin begins to be secreted around this time. But in reality, there are other factors that influence the maturation of the circadian rhythm, and it is more complex than just melatonin.

What about homeostatic sleep pressure? Well, this is a separate mechanism, but closely related. Sleep pressure increases during the hours of wakefulness, and decreases after sleep.[8] When we spend time awake, adenosine builds in the brain and causes us to feel sleepy. Sleep essentially allows the adenosine to drain away, decreasing feelings of sleepiness. This mechanism changes with age, because as you might imagine, babies cannot manage to stay awake for as long as adults. They build up sleep pressure over a shorter time the younger they are.[9] Homeostatic sleep pressure is therefore nothing to do with the circadian rhythm, and increases in response to prior wakefulness. If you haven't been awake long, your sleep pressure is low. If you've been awake for over 18 hours, your sleep pressure will be high. Babies are exactly the same – but for them, their sleep pressure increases at a faster rate, increasing their drive to fall asleep after a shorter period of wakefulness the younger they are.

Overtiredness?

Chances are, you've heard of this concept. Is overtiredness real? Yes – definitely. Is it also overused, over-emphasised, and the cause of a lot of parenting stress? Absolutely. This topic can be viciously debated, with people in some quarters suggesting that overtiredness is wholly overused as a concept, and that you are *never* too tired to sleep. Others claim that overtiredness is the cause of *most* sleep dramas, and the cure for most issues is more sleep, and less awake time. But is the truth actually located somewhere between these two extremes? I think so.

The reasoning for this lies in the fact that the homeostatic sleep pressure and circadian rhythm interact with each other, throughout the day, to determine behaviour over 24 hours. While these two mechanisms are individual, they are more interlinked than many people realise. For example, under very high sleep pressure, there is reduced circadian wake promotion (alertness) – that means that it is easier to fall asleep.[10] This is contrary to the idea that if you are excessively tired, you will not be able to fall asleep. That is not biologically sensible if you think about it. However, being really sleep-deprived causes physiological stress, and stress can increase alertness. In addition, if you stay awake long enough, over-riding your body's tired signals, eventually your circadian rhythm will kick in again and you will feel more alert. Have you ever stayed up all night – either partying 'back in the day', finishing off an essay or studying, or working a night shift? You probably found it is easy to go to sleep quite early in the morning, at say, 7–8am, but by 9.30am, by the time you have had some food, showered and unwound, you may feel really alert, even though the sleep pressure you have built will be even higher. This is your circadian 'wake drive' kicking in. So eventually, because your body clock keeps ticking, whether or not you are asleep, some of those circadian functions will interfere with your sleep pressure right when you don't want them to.

So, it's not true that you can *never* be too tired to sleep, or that being overtired is something you need to worry about on a daily basis. These mechanisms are individual, unique, and affected by other factors. For example, some people who have very active lifestyles seem more resistant to high sleep pressure, or even perform better when they're super tired.[11] For some people, therefore, brain function is adaptive and can adjust to activity levels and sleep pressure.

Some research talks about sleep 'gates' – this is a kind of magic moment, or sweet spot, when you have a sleepy child with high sleep pressure and low circadian wake promotion (alertness). This is when sleep is likely to happen easily. In contrast, if you try to put your child to sleep when they are not tired enough, their sleep pressure is low, and the child is alert,[12] sleep is unlikely to happen easily. This usually happens when a child is either not ready to fall asleep, or has missed their sleep gate and has a 'second wind'.[13] Try and put a child to bed at this time and you're in for a rough ride. You and your child will likely become frustrated and the process will be very drawn out. If this has happened because a nap opportunity was missed, or bedtime was too late, then the best thing to do is relax, don't fight it, and wait for your child to seem calm and sleepy again. If you find this concept difficult because your child's cues are subtle, my suggestion is to not overthink it. The idea that if you miss one single moment to get your child to fall asleep then your whole day will go pear-shaped is a little simplistic. Babies, the sleep process, and our amazing brains are more robust and adaptive than this.

In a similar vein, I hear the phrase 'sleep breeds sleep' nearly every week, either from parents or professionals. But is this true? The short answer is 'not really'. You can only get a certain amount of sleep in 24 hours. The more sleep you get, the lower your sleep pressure will be, and some evidence[14] suggests that the more daytime sleep you get, and the more frequent the naps, the lighter sleep will be – which most certainly does not suggest that sleep breeds sleep. In fact, it suggests the opposite.[15] Of course, there's a balance to be struck. If little ones don't get enough sleep in the day, everyone knows that they can be cranky and miserable and pretty difficult to share life with, but simply recommending more sleep, longer sleep and more frequent sleep is not a blanket answer.

I hope it is now obvious: sleep is not a learned skill. It is a normal homeostatic bodily function. However, it can be and is influenced by habits, our environment, behaviour and sleep hygiene. There is a beautiful sweet spot when it's really easy to fall asleep due to the homeostatic sleep pressure and circadian rhythm being aligned. Sleep pressure builds during the waking hours and is drained away during sleep. But it may be very variable between individuals – recently a gene was discovered that seems to respond to increased brain activity and makes some species sleep more deeply.[16] This may suggest that having a busier brain, or more mental activity in the day, may lead to more catch-up deep sleep – we would need more human studies to be sure, but for now, it's an interesting idea, and one that a lot of people can relate to.

The key message here, when you're thinking about managing the circadian rhythm and sleep pressure, is to create an environment where the two mechanisms are aligned. When sleep pressure is high, and circadian signals are strong, sleep will come more easily, with little to no stress. You do this mainly by exposing your child to plenty of natural light, and observing their natural cues and behaviour. Don't forget that all little ones are different, and prescriptive nap times, even if they work brilliantly for your friend's baby, may not work for your little one at all. Your best bet is to watch your child, and develop an attitude of curiosity about what they need, rather than assuming that all fussy behaviour is due to tiredness.

How are children's sleep states different?

You don't really need to drum this into your head unless you're planning on studying sleep. I'm including this because some parents love to know the science behind sleep. If understanding the science of sleep helps you understand your baby better, then this section is for you. If your eyes start to glaze over with the mention of terms like REM and NREM then skip to 'Why this is not a design fault'. I won't judge you!

There are two basic types of sleep – Rapid Eye Movement (REM) and non-Rapid Eye Movement (NREM). So far, so good. It gets more complicated because there are different stages of NREM sleep – basically going from light sleep (stage 1-2) to deep sleep (stage 3-4). If you're still with me, then take a deep breath, because this is where it gets a bit more complicated. Babies initially go to sleep via REM sleep, and cycle intermittently between REM sleep and stage 3 NREM sleep. Essentially, they have no discernable stage 1-2 NREM sleep (the light sleep). For the committed sleep nerds who are still following me at this point, the infant sleep cycle begins to get a bit interesting around 2-3 months. Around this time, babies begin to have some stage 1-2 sleep, and by about 3-4 months, they go off to sleep via NREM 1-2 sleep, instead of REM.[17,18] If you've followed that – congratulations! Now, why, you might ask, is all this relevant? Well, because the changes to sleep 'architecture' (as it's known in the sleep science world) are related to brain maturity, and have an effect on the length of sleep cycle, and the way babies fall asleep.

Babies' and children's sleep consists of *shorter* sleep cycles – about 50 minutes. The actual type of sleep (REM sleep, light NREM and deep NREM) achieved during these sleep cycles varies with age, but the total length of the sleep cycle remains fairly constant. It lengthens gradually, becoming the more adult-like 90-110 minute sleep cycle by about school age.[19] There are many reasons for this shorter sleep, but one of the most important ones is that babies need to wake frequently to feed.

The second distinct difference between adult and infant sleep is that infants spend more total time in REM (dreaming) sleep. This is crucial for the complex wiring of their brain that occurs during REM sleep. Premature babies' sleep cycles are dominated by REM – which makes a huge amount of sense when you consider that they were born early, and their brain needs even more development and connections to be made. Newborn infants spend at least half their total sleep time in REM sleep.[20] It's easy to tell a baby is in REM sleep – you will see their eyes moving underneath their eyelids, their breathing may be irregular, and they may exhibit some facial twitches, smiles or grimaces. It's actually quite fascinating (and very cute) to watch. Next time you hold a sleeping infant in your arms, or watch them as they nap, know that their brain is literally being built as their eyelids flutter. Remarkably, the parts of the brain that were active during the baby's wakeful time will be active during sleep as well, as the brain processes information and consolidates memory. It's quite profound to watch a baby sleeping once you know this.

The third distinct difference between adult and infant sleep is that infant sleep is fragmented. The official term for this is 'polyphasic' – which means that infants and young children need several periods of alternating sleep and wakefulness, whereas adults generally have a consolidated stretch of nighttime sleep, and a long stretch of wakefulness – known as a monophasic sleep pattern. Not all people in modern cultures have a monophasic sleep pattern. This is most common in Western cultures. Many people in parts of southern Europe and the Caribbean have a biphasic sleep pattern - with a long afternoon nap or siesta, and a consequently later bedtime. People in many parts of Asia and Africa have a polyphasic sleep pattern, with multiple short naps throughout the day, and again, a consequently shorter total nighttime sleep duration.[21] The monophasic sleep pattern is actually a relatively modern (and Westernised) phenomenon, brought about mainly through the invention of the electric light. Before electricity, people went to sleep when it got dark and slept for a few hours. They would typically wake up in the middle of the night and play games, hang out, analyse dreams and do all the other things people do in the middle of the night, and then go back to sleep for another few hours until morning. Nowadays, we have blackout blinds and long hours at work, screens and bright lighting. It's easy to stay up later and we have learnt to adapt to a monophasic sleeping pattern. But just because this is common, doesn't mean that we have always done this.[22,23] In fact, a lot of children fall back into this pattern and are wakeful for a couple of hours in the middle of the night. We are no longer used to this, and find it difficult to handle, but the truth is that this is just your child showing you a behaviour that their ancestors would have had.

Why this is not a design fault

Why children sleep the way they do is a topic of confusion, debate and discussion. There is a large body of research that demonstrates that frequent night waking and feeding is protective against Sudden Infant Death Syndrome (SIDS) and supports optimal feeding.[24-28] If you think about it, waking often is a really sensible idea if you are very small and vulnerable, and need to be kept warm, fed and protected. When babies reach about six months, they begin to experience a different type of brain activity called a K complex. These clever little brain waves suppress the tendency to startle awake to stimuli. This is actually a way of protecting sleep – the brain essentially decides that whatever the noise or other stimulus was, it wasn't important enough to disturb sleep.[29]

Parents often tell me that they would like their infant to sleep more deeply so they don't startle awake to sudden noises. But firstly, we all sleep a little differently. Secondly, you cannot change how deeply a child sleeps unless there is an obvious reason for disruption to their sleep cycle that can be managed with better sleep timing. Finally, you would not want your child to sleep more deeply if it meant they were less safe that way. I know it can be frustrating, but it really isn't a design fault.

We also need to remember that babies are busy adapting to life outside the womb. In utero, they are exposed to maternal sleep hormones and a totally different environment. It's not difficult to see how hard this might be for babies to get used to. Moving from a warm, soft, fluid-filled, sound-muffled, dark and snug place to a bright, loud, cold, and wide-open place can be pretty tough for a little one. We need to remember where babies have come from, and cut them some slack as they learn how to handle the big wide world. This period of adjustment is often referred to as the fourth trimester.[30,31] They will eventually develop their own circadian rhythm. Make their own melatonin. Develop their own ability to regulate their body temperature. But until then, patience is required.

How development affects normal sleep

The other major influence on sleep is development, and this is also not a design fault. Children are constantly growing and changing and adapting. I know this sounds really obvious, and you've seen it with your own eyes, but development really is a global affair. It tends to have knock-on effects on many other areas as well. You might notice your baby is trying really hard to roll, or has just started to belly laugh. They might be managing to get their hands accurately to their mouths, or clap, or sit, or recognise that you've left the room. Whatever it is, it is possible that the cognitive, emotional, social, physical or psychological development that your baby is undergoing will have an effect on sleep. This means that you will notice periods of increased sleep disturbance around times of development. It is almost as if a baby is investing so much energy and thinking power into learning something new that any new habits you are trying to establish with sleep go on hold. The human body is wonderful at prioritising tasks. Learning speech sounds or hand-eye coordination is, on balance, more important than learning that 'Twinkle twinkle little star' means bedtime. I often say to parents that trying to make big changes to sleep during a developmental phase is a little like trying to redecorate while you are having building work done. It's often easier to make changes after the dust has settled.

I can't really go much further without addressing the issue of 'sleep regressions'. No doubt you will have heard of these, or have your own opinion of them. I have an opinion of this term: I hate it. Regression is a word that means a loss or a backward step. In child development, a regression, or the loss of any skill that has previously been demonstrated to have been acquired, is almost always a red flag that requires paediatric evaluation. That is to say it is a term that implies pathology and something 'wrong'. Sleep changes that occur around a time of development are not a sign of something going wrong at all. In fact, this means progress! You will hear people talking with concrete certainty and authority about the 'four-month sleep regression'. This is probably the one that upsets me the most. Sleep changes definitely occur at multiple times during an infant's first year or two, and their development is nearly constant, so it should be obvious that from time to time, sleep is going to be collateral damage. There is actually no evidence at all for a four-month sleep regression. I've looked, I promise. As I mentioned at the beginning of the chapter, there are some pretty massive changes to the way that infants fall asleep, and the proportion of REM to NREM sleep that occurs at some point in the first few months. There is no evidence that it definitely occurs at four months though. Some changes take place around 2–3 months, while others seem to occur at more like 3–4 months. On top of that, there are huge developmental changes that occur at around four months – such as rolling, hand-to-mouth coordination, more vocalisation and so on. Let's also not forget that children who were born slightly early, even if they are not technically preterm, will experience certain neurological changes, including changes to their sleep architecture, at a slightly slower rate. Throw all those variables into the mix, and it might be easier to see why people are so confused about sleep 'regressions'. Clearly, lots of development is going on, and some of that development might impact sleep, but the question is, is it helpful to worry about a sleep 'regression'?

I think not. In my experience, the term causes a lot of unnecessary anxiety, over-pathologising of normal behaviour, and panic that sleep as you know it is about to end completely. The sleep 'regression' that parents may be dreading may never come. Or it may come at a different time. But one thing is for sure: there is nothing you can do about development, and the more you worry about it, the worse it gets. My experience is that when there are some gentle, sensible sleep habits established (more on this in chapter eight), and you prioritise kind, responsive and calm parenting, any changes to sleep will be short-lived and your child will sort themselves out once they've figured out how to giggle, or grab a toy, or go to sleep via NREM – or whatever it is they are currently working on.

Overtired? Bored? Under-stimulated? Wired?

You can't get too far in your Google search for help on baby sleep with-out reading about over-stimulation. I run into polar extremes with this concept depending on which parent or childcare practitioner I am talking to. There is a real danger of making our lives too complicated here. Some babies will be fairly easy-going and able to tolerate lots of stimulation. Others are more content in a quiet, still environment. One study found that children who were more sensitive to environmental stimuli had more trouble falling asleep.[32] There is a certain amount of responsiveness and adaptive parenting that needs to happen here – don't be afraid to watch your baby and see which environments they prefer.

At one extreme, we have the genuinely under-stimulated child. These are children who are never exposed to social situations or different environments, for whom everything is quiet and calm in the home, and excitement is kept to a minimum for fear of over-stimulating the baby. But this is not actually what babies need or want. They *love* social interaction – it's how they learn. They adore different faces, scenes, toys, colours, sounds and lights. It is healthy, natural and normal to maintain normal activities with a baby around, and even to expose them to a wide variety of settings and people.[33] If a baby spends most of their time in a sensory-depleted environment, they can become extremely stressed and sensitive to noises later – there seem to be critical periods when babies need exposure to social interaction and sensory stimuli.[34] Babies need to experience excitement so that they see the ebb and flow of a day. They cannot calm down if they are not excited. Try to give your baby opportunities to laugh, be surprised, excited, and even startled – if they cannot learn about these emotions within the safety of your arms, they will have to learn about them without your help, which is far more stressful. Build in at least one opportunity per day for a different environment, and definitely do not avoid noise and activity around your sleeping baby.

However, the other extreme is the baby who is passed around continuously, never just sitting comfortably on their parent's lap. The baby who is fed by several different people, or the baby who is exposed to music and TV in an effort to intellectually stimulate them. Or the baby who is taken to a different class every day, and swims twice a week. You can have too much of a good thing. This can mean that a baby never has a chance to just observe, be explorative, or interact with people, or you may miss opportunities to observe your baby's cues and facilitate a nap when they are tired. Missing naps can mean your baby becomes cranky.[35] I do meet some overstimulated babies – they either look hyper-alert and 'wired' or start to screech. Your best option if this happens to you is to go somewhere quiet and dark and use movement to help your baby calm down.

So, what's the right kind of stimulation? Well folks, as with so many recommendations, moderation is the key. Your baby will love to go outside, spend time in nature, go swimming, meet animals, see new faces and roll around on the floor exploring. A good rule of thumb is that if you feel overwhelmed, exhausted or have a sense of social overload – your baby probably does too.

Groups are often of huge benefit to parents – and for that reason, I think they are wonderful. They can reduce social isolation and mental health problems, and provide an outlet for parents to offload, get some adult company and receive some support. I remember feeling like activities such as a weekly music class were a lifeline – a chance to see other adults and leave the house. But only go to these groups if you and your baby enjoy them. If they are stressful, find something else. I've met many people who persevere with a baby massage class even when their baby cries through every single one because it's not a good time for them. Don't get me wrong – I love baby massage classes. They're great. I could have picked on baby yoga, or baby sensory, or sing and sign classes. The point is: only do a class if you and your baby find it to be a positive experience. If the time doesn't work – forget it. I'll let you into a secret. If you don't go to any class, ever, your baby won't mind. That's the truth. Your baby will be just as happy doing the grocery shopping in a baby carrier, or sitting in a coffee shop and staring at other babies.

When do children start sleeping through the night?

This question can become like the search for buried treasure. X marks the spot. But what is X? Where is X? And how do you find X? Just like buried treasure, it is often portrayed as the thing that will make all the difference. Well, the truth is that many variables affect sleeping through the night.[36] No one single factor is likely to be the key to unearthing your buried sleep treasure. The myths you may hear about sleeping through the night, and the lived experience of the vast majority of small children and their parents, often bear no resemblance to each other. Of course, some children spontaneously sleep through the night from a very young age and continue with this pattern. Some start sleeping through and then revert to waking up, and some never reliably sleep for long stretches until they are older. Each child will have a different story, and I don't pretend to know yours.

Firstly, how do you define 'sleeping through the night'? Is it 12 hours straight? Is it the hours when *you* would like to be asleep? Or is it just a certain number of hours of continuous unbroken sleep? Research papers define sleep differently, with most using the socially helpful definition of about 10pm–6am.[37] Or is sleeping through the night simply sleep that

> **" One study of over 55,000 children aged 6-18 months found that over 70 percent of them were waking up at least 1-3 times per night. "**

does not disturb the adult? I hear of plenty of parents who bed-share who are unaware of having woken in the night at all. What is the priority? Is it that your baby sleeps for long stretches, or is it that they do not disturb *your* sleep? If you could find a way of quickly and calmly getting back to sleep after attending to your baby, would that be a breakthrough in itself? Every family will have a different priority and objective in their sleep journey. Culture seems to have a significant influence on how you define a sleep problem, what sleeping through the night looks like, and sleep timings.[38]

The fact that children wake up in the night and that this is normal and common is backed up by the research we have available. A UK study of over 700 6-12-month-old babies found that nearly 80 percent woke at least once, and most of them had a feed. The study also found that there was no difference between breast and formula-fed infants.[39] One even larger study of over 55,000 children aged 6-18 months found that over 70 percent of them were waking up at least 1-3 times per night.[40] Only a very small percentage were sleeping through the night. These studies may either depress or reassure you, depending on how old your child is and what your experience has been so far. There is a paradox here, because there are several studies that claim that sleeping through the night can be achieved by three months.[41,42] Firstly though, it is unusual for this behaviour to be spontaneous – for it to be achieved, there is nearly always an intervention. The intervention might include a delayed response, a changed response, or some other intervention.[43] When you do not attempt to modify infant sleep, large-scale studies reveal a different story – worldwide, children rarely sleep through the night, especially not on their own.

The other factor to bear in mind is that *nobody* sleeps all the way through the night. We all stir slightly at the end of every sleep cycle and have no memory of this the next day. Infants and small children have varying abilities to go back to sleep after one of these brief awakenings. The main dialogue in sleep research is whether young children can stop waking their parents up in order to get their help to go back to sleep.[44] Nobody is denying that children wake up numerous times per night. The common desire is for children to stop 'signaling' that they have woken.[45]

Now, some children suck their fingers or thumbs and return to sleep with no help. Others toss and turn and fall back to sleep. Others seem to need more help – these are the children who, in the literature, are diagnosed as having a 'sleep problem'.[46] The goal in many studies therefore is to stop them 'signaling' (crying), so they go back to sleep and do not wake their parents up.[47] The central focus is thus on teaching babies to require less help from their parents in the night – we will come back to this in the next chapter.

Clearly, some children naturally sleep long stretches without any help. Most do not. One study found that about 40 percent of all children were typical sleepers, 45 percent were initially short sleepers but improved, nearly 12 percent were persistent short sleepers and 'poor' sleepers made up 2.5 percent of the sample,[48] but other (larger) studies obviously find that more children take longer than this to consolidate nighttime sleep. Some research suggests that there are certain interventions that can modify night-waking behaviour – but I'm really talking about normal sleep that has not been modified.

There is some suggestion that sleeping for longer stretches at night occurs when the homeostatic process and circadian rhythms are aligned. These processes may both begin at about 2-3 months of age, but they do not necessarily develop at the same time or rate. So it could be that children who sleep through the night earlier have a mature and aligned circadian and homeostatic sleep rhythm that has developed ahead of their peers.[49] We will discuss what gentle interventions you could consider to give sleep a push in the right direction later on, but it is important to get this in perspective – sleeping through the night is a developmental milestone that will be achieved when the child no longer needs a parent's help to fall back to sleep.

When is sleep definitely a problem?

You might be reading this wondering if sleep is *ever* a problem. Although sleep pathology is unusual in babies and young children, it is certainly possible that your child has a condition that needs investigating. Of course, if you are ever unsure, you should ask your doctor or usual healthcare provider. It is a really good idea to keep a diary of symptoms that are bothering you, unusual signs that you have noticed, or sleeping patterns. Video your child if they make strange noises or you are worried about a movement that you see during sleep. The following behaviours or signs all warrant review by a doctor who may want your child to be seen in a specialist clinic:

- Mouth breathing[50]
- Snoring
- Pauses in breathing at night
- Leg or limb movements during sleep that seem or look uncomfortable[51]

Another reason why sleep behaviour may be problematic and require medical help is if your child has a medical condition that affects their sleep. In this case, a sleep problem can be a *symptom* of the underlying condition, not a problem in and of itself. For example, if your child has an allergy, gastro-oesophageal reflux, a cardiac problem, epilepsy, eczema, asthma,[52,53] or other long-term condition, sleep can be affected by their health needs – so you should always check with your doctor if you are unsure. Addressing sleep without figuring out the underlying cause is counter-productive.

Sometimes sleep problems are a symptom of an underlying feeding concern.[54,55] If you are in any doubt, see an International Board Certified Lactation Consultant (IBCLC). Conditions such as tongue-tie,[56,57] wind, mild physiological reflux, shallow attachment (latch), and problems with milk transfer or supply can all manifest as sleep disturbance or problems with settling initially. However, if the underlying cause is feeding-related, then addressing feeding should improve sleep.

Finally, sometimes the reason your sleep situation is so difficult is due to context. There are many difficult contexts I have run into, from bereaved families to older siblings with special or complex needs. If you are finding your sleep situation unworkable, then please see the chapters on optimising child sleep and how to deal with a sleep crisis.

Safe sleep and bed-sharing

Sharing a bed with your baby is an intensely personal decision. The official guidelines steer away from making blanket recommendations in the UK, but in the US, bed-sharing is definitely discouraged.[58,59] But does 'telling' parents not to bed-share mean they won't bed-share? Or does it just make them feel guilty about it and then do it in 'secret' anyway? I firmly believe that most people choose bed-sharing because it is the practical option to get more sleep, and if we do not provide information about it, people will end up doing it anyway, potentially without information about how to make it safer.

I'm not going to tell you to bed-share. I'm also not going to tell you not to. I trust that if you are reading this, you'll be able to make an informed choice about what is best for your family, whether your reasons are related to cuddles and closeness, helping your baby settle better, or simply maximising your own sleep.[60-63] Bed-sharing is not something that is practised in the same way by all families – some try it just in the early days or weeks, while others practise it long-term.[64] Some people claim that bed-sharing can worsen infant sleep. I think that this is a complex situation. Does a parent start to bed-share because they are up so frequently and are trying to maximise their own sleep? Or did the baby only start to feed frequently and wake up more because they were in the bed with their parent? There are hundreds of opinions on this! It is unlikely that bed-sharing is associated with long-term sleep problems. In one large study, bed-sharing and night waking in early infancy were not associated with bed-sharing and night waking in toddlerhood.[65] We also need to remember that bed-sharing is normal and common around most of the world, and has been practised for thousands of years. In countries where bed-sharing is the norm (for example Japan) people tend to have a large, firm mattress, often placed on the floor, and the rates of SIDS are low. Solo-sleeping is actually a relatively modern and western idea, which doesn't fit with many other culturally normal patterns of nighttime parenting.

If you are planning to share a bed with your baby, the current recommendations are: [66,67]

- Babies should always sleep on their back
- Choose a firm sleep surface
- Babies should sleep in the same room as parents
- Avoid smoking (including passive smoking), alcohol and drugs
- Breastfeed if you can, for as long as you can
- Immunisation seems to protect infants (though that is a whole other conversation)
- Skin-to-skin contact at birth
- Avoid baby sleep positioners, teddies, and other objects in the bed

- Never bed-share if you or your partner smoke, take drugs (including prescription drugs which make you sleepy, such as antihistamines and painkillers), if you are extremely tired, or your baby was born prematurely or is very small
- Never fall asleep with your baby on a chair or sofa
- If your baby has been using a dummy/soother/pacifier, then do not suddenly stop it if your baby is under six months old

That's a long list! It is not always easy to make an informed decision, as the studies that are available so far haven't always separated out risk factors that are known to increase SIDS risk (such as sleeping on a sofa, smoking and so on) from families who have followed all the recommendations.[68-70] Therefore, it is difficult to say for sure whether bed-sharing increases the risk of SIDS.[71] One study found a very small increase in risk when researchers controlled for families in which nobody smoked and the baby was breastfed,[72] but on the whole, the consensus from many researchers is that there is insufficient evidence to suggest that bed-sharing increases the risk of SIDS.[73]

It is also important to say that some people start off bed-sharing and then want to move on from it. Bed-sharing can be a flexible arrangement if you want, and you can also decide to stop later on if it is no longer working for you. There are some ideas about how to stop bed-sharing with love in the chapter on how to deal with a sleep crisis.

The tired parent's summary

- Most infants and children have no sleep pathology.
- Everyone's unique circadian rhythm influences sleep and this can be shaped by social cues, noise, activity and especially natural light exposure.
- Sleep pressure builds during waking time and increases the drive to fall asleep. It is independent of the circadian rhythm.
- Trying to get a child to fall asleep when their sleep pressure is low (they are not tired enough) or high (they are over-tired) is harder. Observing your individual child for their optimal awake windows and sleep gates leads to less frustration and better sleep.
- Everyone has cycles of sleep. Babies' sleep cycles are initially shorter and simpler, developing, maturing and increasing in complexity as they get older.

- The ways in which infant sleep is different may sometimes feel frustrating, but it is the way it is for many good reasons - mostly related to infant safety.
- During normal developmental stages, sleep can change and become more fragmented.
- Babies expect, benefit from and require stimulation, play, social interaction, nature time and changes of scene. There is a balance to be had between doing too much and too little.
- Sleeping 'through the night' is a highly variable developmental stage, affected by many factors - many of which are outside individual parental control.
- For the minority of babies and children who do have sleep pathology such as periodic limb movement disorder or sleep apnoea, medical evaluation and intervention is required.
- Bed-sharing is often part of the safe sleep dialogue. Bed-sharing is normal in many cultures, and 'telling' parents not to utilise a tool that makes the nighttime easier may not be the best approach.
- Making decisions about sleep location is highly personal, and needs to be individualised so that important risk factors are recognised and any risks are minimised.

Chapter seven

Naps

How is daytime sleep different from nighttime sleep? Isn't sleep just sleep? Well, dear reader, the short answer is no. Nap sleep has a different function, and is structured differently.[1] Do you remember that infants have polyphasic sleep? The reason for this is that initially, with little to no circadian control of sleep, babies just sleep on and off throughout the 24-hour period, largely driven by hunger, sleep pressure and the need to feed frequently, as well as their short sleep cycle.

Babies begin making their own melatonin any time from 1-6 months, but usually by about three months. If your baby is being breastfed, then your milk contains a hormone called tryptophan, which is used by your body to make melatonin, so a breastfed baby will get a little bit of help,[2] but they still won't make their own sleep hormone initially. This means in practice that there is just as much sleep occurring in the day, and no long stretches occurring at night.[3] Once they achieve circadian rhythmicity (knowing their days from their nights), you will probably notice more awake time in the day rather than at night, which is when naps might begin to look distinct, or even develop a tiny bit of predictability.

It isn't all about babies' circadian rhythm though. Naps do not just evolve because of an established circadian rhythm. They also change because little ones cannot stay awake as long as an older child or adults. The amount of time they can stay awake varies with age and has individual variability. Naps function to take the edge off your baby or toddler's tiredness. It really is that simple. This is why you may notice that as a newborn your baby sleeps on and off all day and night, whereas as they get older, you will notice distinct periods of wakefulness and activity in between sleep periods in the daytime. The length of these bouts of wakefulness will increase over time.

The effect of missed naps

Some studies have shown that naps help to reduce the cortisol that builds as we become more tired. You might remember from the previous chapter that as sleep pressure builds, infants (like all of us!) can get cranky and stressed. Without a chance to release some of that sleep pressure with a nap, a baby or young child is like a pressure cooker with too much steam. Releasing the pressure at periodic intervals reduces the stress and keeps your baby happier in the daytime.[4] It sounds great in theory, doesn't it? But you may need to accept a little trial and error with getting the timings right for *your* baby. All babies are different. There is also *some* evidence[5-9] that not enough sleep in the day can have the following effects:

- Shorten the sleep cycle
- Shorten the duration of sleep
- Make sleep more fragmented
- Cause early rising
- Lead to fussy, cranky behaviour or hyperactivity

You may notice other signs as well - since you are the world expert on your child, you'll be the best person to say how a missed nap affects your little one. Research studies aside, from a parental perspective, most people find that a skipped nap means a cranky child, a disrupted evening, or difficult behaviour. For parents, naps are also a chance for you to decompress, have some time out, or sleep - so I totally understand why nap dramas are so frustrating.

How many naps?

Have you ever asked Google this question? You will find hundreds of blogs, tables and charts suggesting how many naps your baby needs at different ages. I even included one in my previous book. But these charts need to be taken with a big grain of salt. They are based on large studies that look at how many hours of sleep most children achieve in a 24-hour period, and many of the studies differentiate between daytime sleep and nighttime sleep.[10-12] So far so good. However, no study that I am aware of has examined *how long an infant can be awake for* at different ages. I am actually quite grateful for this. It means (at least in theory) that parents should exercise their own judgement and superior knowledge of their child to determine an individual rhythm that works for their child, which will of course change with age. There is not even a lot of data about how many naps a child should have – most books and blogs are based on observation and clinical experience. One study found that most infants under six months have at least two naps per day, and by 18 months, most infants are napping just once.[13] That isn't actually a lot of information to go on though, and many people find their babies need more naps than this. It also isn't just about the number of naps, but also the length of naps – about which, again, there is very little available evidence.

The number of naps your child has will depend on how long they can tolerate being awake in between. Different children show different signs of being tired. Your child may whine, fuss, rub their eyes, or yawn. Or they may do none of those things. You will have to watch them and notice their behaviour before they fall asleep. I know that doesn't sound very scientific, but if you learn to be attuned to your baby's behavioural cues, you will quickly notice when they are telling you they need a rest.

Because there is no concrete data about this, I can only give you a rough idea based on experience. Please know, however, that this may look wildly different for your baby. It is intended as a loose guide only – if it causes you anxiety or stress then ignore it! Also remember that if your baby was born prematurely you will need to adjust your expectations.

Age	Total sleep in 24 hours	Total hours of daytime sleep	Total hours of nighttime sleep	Number of naps	Approximate awake time between naps
Birth to 6 weeks	14-17	Variable	Variable	Evenly spread	30-60 minutes
6-12 weeks	14-17	Variable	Variable	6-7	60-75minutes
3-4 months	13-15	4-5	9-10	4-6	1.25-1.75 hrs
4-5 months	13-15	4-5	9-10	3-4	1.5-2.25 hrs
5-6 months	13-15	4-5	9-10	3	1.5-2.5 hrs
6-7 months	12-14	3-4	10-11	3	2-2.75 hrs
7-8 months	12-14	3-4	10-11	2-3	2.25-3 hrs
8-9 months	12-14	3-4	10-11	2-3	2.5-3.5 hrs
9-10 months	11-14	2-3	10-11	2	3-4 hrs
10-12 months	11-14	2-3	10-11	2	3.5-4.5 hrs
12-16 months	11-14	2-3	10-11	2	4-6 hrs
16-24 months	11-14	2-3	10-11	1	5-7 hrs

When to drop naps?

Having invested a lot of time and effort into getting naps going, there will come a day when you'll think about when to ditch them. You may want to drop a nap because it's being resisted. Or your child may simply not need as many (or any) naps. If your child gets less sleep in total on a nap day than they do without a nap, then they are ready to drop it. For example, if your three-year-old has a two-hour nap, but is then three hours later for bed, there is a net loss of one hour of sleep in 24 hours. So it would be sensible to drop the nap. But if you find that with a nap, your child gets more sleep in 24 hours or the same amount of sleep, then it is worth continuing it. For example, if your three-year-old has a one-hour nap and is one hour later to bed, it is still worth having the nap, as the nap is probably preventing a cranky afternoon.

It is not uncommon for a nap to be dropped in the hope that this will make bedtime easier. What often happens when a child is prevented from napping is that they are so exhausted that they fall asleep very quickly. This is frequently interpreted as a success. But crashing out like this *can* sometimes backfire if your child was very fatigued, and can lead to more night waking.

For example:

Dylan is two years old. He started nursery recently and has been very busy in the day. He began to have shorter midday naps a few weeks ago. Soon afterwards, his parents found that he was difficult to get to bed at bedtime. They noticed that if he didn't nap at all, or had a very short (less than 30-minute) nap, he would fall asleep faster at bedtime. This led them to believe that Dylan's nap was causing the bedtime battle. He then started waking up earlier in the morning. In turn this led to him being more fatigued earlier in the evening and they started an earlier bedtime.

In this (very common) scenario, it is easy to see the logic: less sleep in the day equals faster, easier bedtime. It is also easy to understand how some people can associate early rising with a decreased need for overall night-time sleep, and cut this short by delaying bedtime. However, the easier bedtime is often a temporary change. Sometimes a sleep debt can take some time to build.

What actually happened was that Dylan still needed that nap. The loss of the nap is resulting in a vicious circle of fatigue and crankiness, and both the lack of nap and late bedtime are resulting in early rising. The solution is to carve out protected time for the nap, minimise distractions, create a calm sleep space, and also remember that he may need more time for connection with his parents, having recently started nursery. If they persevere with an earlier bedtime, this reduces the availability of connection time. But also, it is unrealistic to expect a child of two to achieve more than about 11 hours of sleep, so the early bedtime may reinforce early rising. Reinstating the nap makes it more likely that Dylan will make it through to a bedtime that acknowledges a normal 11 hours of overnight sleep without waking up at 5am.

While I run into a few toddlers who genuinely don't seem to need a nap, it is a sensible strategy to assume that *most* do. You'll know your toddler is ready to drop their nap entirely when:

- They sleep well at night
- They are generally cheerful (I don't mean *all* the time – everyone is allowed to have a bad day, or a bad reaction!)
- They settle relatively easily for bed at night, with no apparent hyperactivity

If you can't be sure of these factors, then the likelihood is your toddler is not ready to abandon their nap just yet. Sometimes a toddler will need an *occasional* nap – perhaps every few days, or after a particularly busy day. It doesn't have to be all or nothing.

For many families, the loss of the nap is mourned not only for the effect on the rest of the day, but also because the parent doesn't get that time to recharge their batteries and have a break. Toddlers are hard work, and it's totally normal to need a break and some space. It really helps if you model the need for blank space in the day to relax, unwind and just *be*. As a society, we are getting less and less adept at being still, being bored and just existing. Filling every moment with activity, stimulation, connectedness to the outside world and rapid thought is exhausting, and ultimately not particularly good for us. We all need space to decompress. Encourage your child to have a quiet time of playing, looking at books, listening to an audiobook on their bed, or sitting in a den or cave while listening to meditation tracks. This is really important and has been shown to reduce stress, even if sleep is not achieved.[14]

One final thought – sometimes parents are not sure whether dropping a nap is a good idea or not. Occasionally I run into children where there doesn't seem to be a good option. For example, having a nap means a cheerful afternoon but a difficult bedtime, or not having the nap means a cranky afternoon but an easy bedtime. Sometimes you have to pick the lesser of two difficult situations! Some hybrid options include:

- A very short power nap of just 10-15 minutes
- Napping on alternate days
- An earlier bedtime
- Condensing two naps into one - for example, making a morning nap later and an afternoon nap earlier until they are one and the same

Don't be afraid to experiment and try things out. Eventually you'll find a pattern that works for you.

What about nap 'refusal'?

Nap dramas can be particularly frustrating because skipping a nap can mean an unbearably cranky little person towards the end of the day. There are numerous reasons why napping might have become so difficult.

Developmental changes

It is not going to make headlines that developmental changes at any age can affect sleep. Children develop across different areas, often at different times. Sometimes these changes occur all at the same time. A burst of language development, along with increasing physical gross motor skills, and an increased sense of autonomy, may all coincide. When children are in the throes of major developmental change, sleep is often collateral damage. Life is simply a bit too confusing, or exciting, or frustrating, or scary, or all of those things at the same time, to sleep.

Too many exciting things going on in the day

It can be hard to get the balance right between getting out and about, seeing people and getting chores done, and having quiet time. There are lots of classes for babies and toddlers, and they sometimes force a change in routine which means nap time gets squeezed. I remember booking a swimming class for my youngest daughter that was perfectly timed at the beginning of the block of lessons, but by the end of them, her nap patterns had changed, and she really didn't cope well with the swim class! Of course, these things are often a) unavoidable and b) temporary.

Separation anxiety

For babies approaching 7-9 months, separation anxiety can cause some sleep and settling difficulty. In toddlers, their new-found independence and increased autonomy is exciting, but also scary. It is not unusual for them to struggle to switch off at naptime, or to suddenly not want to be left alone.

Return to work, or a major change in dynamic

There may be some major changes, particularly if your baby is older. You may return to work, or another sibling may come along. These factors do not in and of themselves cause sleep disruption, but the change in routine or environment may cause nap problems.

A badly timed car trip

This is a really common problem, and doesn't only apply to car rides, but also to pushchairs/strollers. If your child has a 5-10 minute doze in the car or pushchair on the way back from a school run, or an errand, then what basically happens is that they have enough sleep to lift the lid on that pressure cooker, and sleep pressure falls slightly. This can be enough to mean that the nap (or bedtime) is entirely refused as the sleep pressure won't be quite high enough to have a fully restorative nap. If this seems to be the pattern, either prolong the nap, or try to change the way or time the errand happens so that the child does not fall asleep at an inopportune time. For example, allow older toddlers to ride their scooter to the shop rather than putting them in the pushchair. Turn them around in the baby carrier so they are more visually stimulated. Or offer snacks to keep them busy. Both of my children turned me into a fan of taking the bus rather than using the car, as they were prone to having a crafty five-minute car sleep which would mean game over at bedtime.

FOMO (fear of missing out)

Many babies, and especially toddlers, are resistant to taking a nap because there are far more exciting things to do. They don't want to leave the action in order to go to sleep – which seems infinitely less interesting than whatever is going on around them.

Overtiredness

While overtiredness can be an overused term, this is especially likely if your child has just dropped a nap and the problems began shortly after the nap was dropped. What sometimes happens is that a nap is dropped (appropriately) and your child develops some sleep debt during the course of the day. The next nap time may need to be altered to compensate. What often happens is that if the nap is too *early*, there is not *enough* sleep pressure, and the child either refuses the nap altogether, or it is very short. If the nap is too *late*, there is too *much* sleep pressure, and your child becomes wired and will typically refuse their nap.

How to help a reluctant napper

There are many ways to help your little one if they clearly still need a nap. Consider the following ideas:

Give more autonomy to your child

Sometimes a good old-fashioned rebrand helps! Call it quiet time, calm-down time, snooze time, or down-time, if the word 'nap' sends your toddler running for the back garden. Or try reverse psychology: 'I know you're not tired right now, but let's sit and snuggle for 10 minutes on your bed'. It's worth a go.

Altering timings

Going from two naps to one can be particularly hard. If the first nap has recently been abandoned, try the midday nap slightly earlier temporarily, and also an earlier bedtime to compensate for a) fatigue and b) the earlier nap timing. As the sleep debt is caught up, what you may find is that your child begins to wake earlier in the morning. If and when this happens, make the nap and bedtime later again to get back on track.

Consider flexibility

It doesn't have to be all or nothing. On a sedentary day, a nap may be less needed, and on a mentally challenging or physically tiring day it may be more needed. Or a sleep debt may be subtle and only build up over several days. A nap every few days may suit your child. Also consider being flexible about the location of the nap. For some children, total elimination of distractions may be necessary, whereas for others, a strategic push-chair nap or car ride at the right time can facilitate the nap happening rather than being skipped entirely. Car naps are not a long-term strategy, but they are better than no nap at all, and can get the nap habit back in place again.

Try a change of scene

It may be necessary to relocate to somewhere quieter and less stimulating. Outdoors is a great place to try this. Spread a rug under a tree, read some books and see if your child will take a nap outdoors. Or put a yoga mat under the kitchen table and cover the table with a thick dark blanket. Your child may have a nap in this dark, quiet 'cave'.

Eliminate distractions

It is possible to maintain alertness and stave off fatigue by using distractions, food, activities and screens. These are often instigated to ward off tantrums and irritability caused by tiredness, or prevent a poorly timed nap! Consider whether you are beginning to use food and activities to manage behaviour that could be managed with sleep instead. Some parents find a diary helps to spot this pattern. Of course, you know your child best – if you have found that a nap is not what your child needs, or it will cause a bedtime backfire, then by all means head outdoors, dance around, or snuggle on the sofa instead.

Ensure plenty of exercise and mental stimulation

Toddlers have a lot of energy and their brains are constantly busy. They should rarely just be sitting still without moving their bodies. Plan for plenty of time for them to be busy. Toddlers love to be given jobs to do, so break down jobs into numerous parts and that will keep them busy and active for longer. It won't occur to them that there is a more efficient way of completing a task! Also plan time for them to run, jump, chase, walk, skip, hop, cycle and bounce. In between periods of activity, plan activities that make them think. Try burying toys in plasticine for them to find, or consider simple jigsaw puzzles or shape-sorters. Hide toys around the house and ask the toddler to find the 'red ball', the 'blue bag', the 'green spoon'. Ask them to find 'three things that are circle-shaped'. You'll be helping them to problem-solve, think, persevere, and learn language as well as move about – all while you get to sit down and maybe drink some hot coffee.

Prioritise a calm-down time

Just as important as activity level is strategically planning in a few minutes of distinct calm-down time prior to a nap or bedtime. If your child is excited, a short pre-sleep routine may not be enough to get them calm. Dim the lights, soften and lower your voice, maybe try some yoga together, and reduce distractions even before you enter the sleeping space (wherever that is). You'll stand a better chance of making that much-needed nap happen.

Thinking about naps one step at a time

I have found that people often become frustrated by their nap situation. Maybe you are currently rocking or feeding your baby to sleep. Perhaps the only way your little one will sleep is being driven in the car, or pushed in the pushchair/pram/stroller. Whatever it is, the chances are you're doing it that way because it is the quickest, easiest, or most reliable way of getting your little one to sleep. May I suggest you take the pressure off yourself? Give yourself permission to *not* address everything all at the same time. Breaking a daunting task into manageable steps is a good psychological hack that makes problems feel more manageable. I often share these four steps to sleep:

1. You can get your child to sleep at a time that works for them, using any means necessary, in any location that will work
2. You can get your child to sleep at a time that works for them, using any means necessary, with some limits on location that work for you
3. You can get your child to sleep at a time that works for them, using any means necessary, in the location that works for you
4. You can get your child to sleep at a time that works for them, with the support and location that works for you

If you're currently struggling to get the timing of naps right for your child, then there's very little point in beating yourself up about the fact that you rely on the baby carrier to get your little one to sleep. Work on getting the timings right first, then see what other small changes you can make. For example:

Fox is an 11-month-old little boy whose parents struggle to get him to nap anywhere except the pushchair. They have persevered with cot naps, but Fox ends up refusing to nap at all, and becomes cranky. Step 1 was to be observant of Fox's individual cues for boredom, tiredness or other factors. Fox was then taken out in the pushchair in the morning and again after lunch, with a predictable mini version of his bedtime routine before the walk in the pushchair. This went on for a couple of weeks. Then, for step 2 they did the same, but instead of continuous motion, they began parking the pushchair under a tree and swaying it only very slightly, and the pushchair was also reclined fully. Step 3 for Fox meant putting him in the pushchair, walking a short distance, then bringing the pushchair into the house to finish the nap off. Fox's parents initially had just the last 10 minutes of his nap in the house, and worked up to longer periods indoors. Step 4 was to replicate the routine they had developed, but lie down with Fox on a mattress on the floor, cuddling him while he fell asleep. Fox's parents then slowly inched away from him as he became used to the changes.

Does location matter?

Many people ask where their baby should sleep. I think this is ultimately your choice. Most studies focus on where an infant should sleep at night, or discuss this from the SIDS perspective of keeping infants near their parents for all sleep episodes for safety purposes.[15] I often hear people saying that sleep routines and locations need to be 100 percent consistent so that babies will sleep 'better'. But is there any actual evidence that this is true? You guessed it – no. There are lots of anecdotal tales, but no scientific evidence to back it up. So, we are stuck with using common sense. Should your baby or child nap in a pushchair or stroller? A baby carrier? In your arms? At your breast/chest? In a crib/cot? Be wary of anyone who tells you something prescriptive about nap location. You will hear that naps always need to be at home, in the crib, in the dark, for example. Let's unpack that for a moment. The premise with this advice is that babies will sleep longer, more reliably, and get into a habit of taking these naps. What is the flip side though? I would argue that needing to nap in the dark, at home, in the quiet is restrictive and prevents you from getting out of the house, from having company, and may increase social isolation, boredom and anxiety. Another issue is that your baby may become so accustomed to napping with these environmental cues that they lose the ability to be adaptable. Who wants to have to rush home from a really fun day out because otherwise their child won't nap? Or cut a long leisurely lunch short because there is no way the baby can nap in a restaurant with ambient noise and light? I would urge you to maintain flexibility for your own sanity, and your baby's adaptive behaviour.

What about the fear that babies will not develop healthy sleep habits if they do not always nap in their crib or cot? Or that nap location must mirror nighttime sleep location? I think we do babies a disservice to assume that they cannot be flexible. I have never met a baby who cannot nap in one way, and achieve nighttime sleep in another. They are capable of discerning between different contexts – go back to your step-wise approach to working on naps. If you're still stuck at step 1, there's no point trying to move on to step 4.

Sometimes naps are a logistical or practical problem rather than an actual sleep issue. Everyone has days when napping on the run is a reality. Errands have to get done, nursery and school runs need to happen. Then you add mealtimes into the mix and it can get quite tricky to fit in a nap. Again, think about addressing just one aspect of your child's nap situation at a time. Only work on what you can realistically change, and don't forget, just like every other aspect of sleep – it's only a problem if it's a problem for you.

If you choose to work on naps...

If you are keen to make one nap consistent, you could either go for the nap that is the easiest to achieve, or the longest, or the one that is likely to be dropped the last. One practical suggestion is that if you're going to try something new (like a cot nap), or potentially difficult, do not try it at a nap that has historically been difficult to achieve – you are probably setting yourself and your little one up for a difficult time. If the first nap is always guaranteed, try the difficult thing then – it has the best chance of success.

I like to encourage parents to think about what the best nap *for their family* to work on might be, rather than telling them which one. For example, you might have real difficulty getting naps to happen anywhere but the baby carrier, but have found that the first nap of the day is the most reliable one. Great – work on that one.

Having said that, if you have a nursery or school run around the time of your baby's first nap, then there's probably no point in making this a home nap. Instead, think about which one will be easiest given your other commitments. The lunchtime nap might be the one you want to get right, since for most children this is the last nap to be dropped. Or if you have two napping children, you might want to try to work on a synchronised nap. Whatever works for you is a good place to start.

One last thought – sometimes the driving force to change a nap is you. That's okay too! Here are some common examples I run into:

- Wanting to stop pushchair naps because the weather is terrible, and you don't enjoy the rigidity of having to go for a walk just to achieve a nap
- Needing to stop using a baby carrier for naps because you are pregnant, and your bump is getting too big/baby is getting heavy
- Being forced to stop rocking to sleep because of back problems
- Choosing to stop feeding to sleep because of a return to work

There are as many reasons for wanting to change nap logistics as there are families. If the sleep situation isn't working for you, it's okay to want to change it. There are plenty of ways to do that with love and respect.

Short naps? Long naps?

The length of your child's nap may be another source of confusion and stress. Some sleep experts say that short naps are not restorative, while others say that they are normal and just related to individual body rhythms and sleep needs. So, there is some controversy here. I tend to take a pragmatic view. If your child appears cranky when they wake from their nap, then it is possible that they woke prematurely. If they are perfectly happy and seem well rested, and nothing else is wrong with their nights, then I would not worry about it. I appreciate that often our desire for our child to take a longer nap is related to our own need to have some time out, get jobs done, work or sleep ourselves, but there is very little you can do to make a child sleep more than they need to. Some research suggests that the amount and type of sleep you achieve depends on the number of nap opportunities. So, if you have multiple naps, you sleep lightly, and if you just have one nap, your sleep is deeper. [16] If your baby is a short napper, it is likely they will need more nap opportunities to prevent them from becoming overtired, but that isn't to say that this is a negative outcome.

Sometimes, long naps come once a child is more physically active. Sometimes it is related to development. Sometimes it appears to be genetic. You may find that your little one finally starts to take a long nap at midday once they are walking, or otherwise getting more active. Often, parents report that their children sleep better after a swimming lesson. Experiment with different locations as well. If you find that your baby or toddler naps for a long period when they are close to you – in the baby carrier or lying next to you on a bed – but sleep for a short time in their crib or pushchair, then it is likely that the short nap is related to location, rather than their unique biorhythm. If this is the case, work on the timing of the nap, in the location where sleep is longest (step 1), and once it is more habituated, you could then begin to make some changes to the location.

A word of warning about 'longer' naps. Because there is only so much sleep that a child can achieve in the day, if they have really long naps, you might find that the trade-off is a more fragmented night, or even a party in the night – known commonly as a 'split night'. What often happens is that if your naps are long and bedtime is relatively early, by the time your little one has slept 5-6 hours, they may have had most of the sleep they need in 24 hours. They sometimes then wake up at 1-2am and stay awake for a couple of hours. You might remember that this was normal until the widespread use of the electric light, but nowadays it is pretty inconvenient if your little one does this. Usually, applying logic helps. If you count up how many hours of sleep in 24 hours your child is likely to need, and subtract the number of hours of sleep they get in the day, the answer may be staring you in the face. For example:

Marta was a five-month-old baby, who was a spectacular napper, taking three 90-minute naps per day, and then happily going to bed at 7pm. However, she was awake from midnight until 2am, as well as having regular wake-ups in the night. This rhythm had been in place since Marta was 10 weeks old, but in the last six weeks Marta has been having split nights.

For this baby, 13-15 hours of sleep in 24 hours is a reasonable expectation. But she's achieving 4.5 hours of sleep in the day, which leaves only 8.5 hours at night at the lower end of the total sleep estimate. That means that if this family don't want to start their day any earlier than 6am, bedtime would realistically need to be 9.30pm. The alternative is that they shorten Marta's naps in the day, so that she's getting closer to three hours of sleep in the day. The point is that sometimes there is a choice to be made between prioritising daytime sleep and nighttime sleep.

Nap rhythms

Finally, you may hear about some napping patterns that are related to the time of day. Some of the patterns I hear about are:

- Short - long - short
- The 2, 3, 4 nap pattern

I really believe that most families will find a pattern that works for them, and in general, I'm not a fan of scheduling naps, or prescribing a set pattern. I'll explain a bit more about these patterns and you can make up your own mind.

The short-long-short pattern is for babies who take three naps. The idea is to top up a baby's sleep in the morning, but not give them too long a nap first thing. The theory behind this is that if they have a long nap in the morning they might then not be tired enough for a nap in the middle of the day. If they skip that, or it's late, they may only end up with two naps and a cranky afternoon. The third nap is important for many babies to prevent a very crabby baby during the late afternoon and before bedtime.

The 2, 3, 4 nap pattern, in my experience, only works for a very small number of babies, for a very short window of time. But if you find it works for your little one - the good news is that it's pretty easy to remember! You put them down for their first nap *two* hours after first waking, put them down for their second nap *three* hours after waking from the first one, and put them to bed *four* hours after waking from the second. For example, if your baby woke at 6am, nap one would be 8am, then assuming this nap is an hour, nap two would be at 12pm, and assuming that nap is 2.5 hours, you would start bedtime at 6.30pm. The reason it only works for a small number of babies is that it relies on fairly long naps, which not all children manage to achieve. It also only works if they are both content with just two naps, and can also go back to sleep just two hours after waking. Like I said, if it's working for you, that's awesome, but if you happen to have googled it and tried it, only to find it was a disaster – don't worry. Just ditch it.

What about that big taboo - waking children from naps? Never wake a sleeping baby, right? Or should you? You will have to be guided by your own little one here. But there are some situations when it's the right thing to do. For example, if your baby has a very long morning nap and then it messes up the rest of your day. Or if they have a late nap, and you know that this means a bedtime battle. Finally, as I've already mentioned, too much daytime sleep can lead to a split night. It's okay to wake your child from their nap if you feel this is the right thing in context.

I want to throw a curveball to finish with here. You are not a renegade if there is no pattern to your child's naps. It is totally legitimate to simply go with the flow and allow your child to nap on the run, whenever they seem to need to nap. This may sound a little radical, but actually, this is how babies sleep all over the world, and for thousands of years. Simply not overthinking your child's naps, and going with it, can take the pressure off, increase spontaneity, and reduce anxiety. Just a thought.

The relationship between naps and nights

Several studies have shown that naps and nighttime sleep are related. One Icelandic study found that the timing of daytime sleep influences the quality of nighttime sleep. To optimise sleep, the amount of time between the last nap and bedtime should be increased to four hours of awake time if they had two naps, and 5-6 hours of awake time if they had one nap.[17] Another study in Japan agreed that an afternoon nap tends to delay sleep onset at night.[18] One systematic review consistently found across several papers that napping in the day is associated with less sleep at night - especially after the age of two years.[19] This is not really a surprise - after all, you can only get so much sleep in 24 hours, so it has to even out somewhere. There is a critical balance between getting enough sleep and getting too much at the 'wrong' time. It would be nice if we could honestly say that the more sleep you get in the day the more sleep you'll get at night, but there is obviously a limit to the truth of this statement. Another study of nearly 4,000 three-month old Thai babies found that napping more than three times in the day is associated with more nighttime awakening.[20]

Great naps, bad nights? It could be that your child is having too much sleep in the day, or the sleep is not well-timed. Try experimenting with different timings, locations, or even wake your baby a little earlier to see if this helps. It could be that an earlier night might help as well.

Bad naps, good nights? You may need to examine your expectations about what a 'good nap' looks like. If your child is a short napper and is perfectly happy and sleeping well at night, then it is likely that this is their natural body rhythm. However, if they are cranky in the day and seem unhappy, then you might have more luck with less time awake in between naps. Play around with timings until your child seems more rested and content in the daytime.

Bad naps, bad nights? First of all, you may want to review how much sleep your little one is achieving. It may be that it is actually within the normal range, and acceptance is what is needed. Or there could be an underlying problem with discomfort, gas, a feeding issue, or a health problem. If this is a new problem, perhaps your child's sleep needs have changed. Would fewer or shorter naps help? If your little one has always slept like this, then perhaps the entire day needs an overhaul. Review your little one's awake times, and bedtime, and see the chapter on sleep optimisation in babies.

So, despite a lack of research on daytime napping structure, organisation and implementation, I have some general suggestions for you:

- Naps are highly variable. Observe your baby closely and see what works for them with regard to the amount of time they can tolerate being awake between naps
- Newborns nap on and off all day and night. This gradually morphs into a pattern of more sleep at night by about 2-3 months
- In general, you can expect a baby under six months to have at least 2-3 naps
- You can expect a baby between 6-18 months to need two naps
- You will probably see your toddler of 18 months only needing one nap
- Naps are usually dropped completely by somewhere between 2-4 years
- Consider a flexible approach to location of naps
- The length of your child's naps is also highly variable

Chapter eight

Night feeds

→ I wonder how many times you have heard or read about night feeding in the context of sleep? Have you been asked whether your child is 'still' feeding in the night? Have you searched for answers about this on the internet? Have you heard of feeding to sleep being labelled a sleep association/crutch? How does that make you feel?

The truth is, babies and children wake up in the night for multiple different reasons (just like you and me) – but feeding is a big one, so we tend to hang all our hopes on them stopping night feeding in order to sleep for longer stretches. But is this realistic? If they stop waking to feed will they stop waking full stop? Or does this just eliminate one of many reasons why children wake up? How do we separate feeding for hunger and feeding for comfort and as a tool to aid sleep? At what point is it reasonable to put some limits on night feeds? So many questions and, I'll be honest with you – a lot of conflicting and confusing information.

Modifying practices such as feeding to sleep, and night feeds, usually comes up as a strategy to attempt to improve sleep. Many sleep research articles and textbooks suggest that infants do not need night feeds after six months.[1] But who says they are not necessary? At what point does feeding to sleep become perceived as problematic? And is this a holistic way to think about infant care? Let's explore these tricky issues in more depth.

The premise is that if a night feed is not necessary after six months, then continuing them:

a) is unnecessary
b) is therefore about comfort, or habit
c) may self-perpetuate night waking, and
d) could theoretically reduce daytime appetite

Firstly, are night feeds necessary after six months?

Several papers and well-known paediatric sleep textbooks suggest that night feeds are unnecessary after six months. However, they do not explain *why* they are unnecessary beyond the idea of feeding becoming a 'sleep association'. They do not provide any clinical justification for night feeds being unnecessary at this age, or explain what is different between five months and six months that marks this change. Finally, none of these papers or textbooks are written by infant feeding experts. They are coming at this problem from a behavioural sleep perspective, and so perhaps are not the best people to be discussing normal trajectories of infant feeding and nighttime behaviours. Textbooks discussing night feeds after six months assume that this is a problematic behaviour. But what if it is just normal?

I cannot find any consistent rationale for the idea that night feeds are unnecessary after six months. Some studies have noticed a drop-off in night feeding after six months, although this is not consistent, and other studies find that night waking increases after six months. It could also be related to infants eating solid food by this point. But starting solids has not been shown in large, well-designed studies to improve nighttime sleep, or to reduce the need to feed at night.[2] The other explanation for the potential lack of necessity of night feeds may be related to infants being able to last longer between feeds. But what is the big physiological difference between a five-month-old baby and a six-month-old baby? This may not be a generalisable statement across all babies, and may also fail to account for differences in appetite, metabolism and individual caloric need.

Some very large studies exploring night-feeding behaviours in infants disagree with the idea that night feeds are unnecessary after six months.[3,4] In fact, one study looked at night-waking patterns of over 55,000 babies aged 6–18 months and found that 70 percent of them woke on average 1–3 times, mostly needing a night feed.[5] Other smaller studies find that there are two distinct groups of sleeping pattern, and that while most babies sleep through the night at six months, babies with a 'higher need' temperament were more likely to wake at night and need feeding.[6]

Another aspect worth considering is that if night feeds are stopped, is this likely to have an adverse impact on breastfeeding duration and milk supply? One study found that discouraging parents from night feeds was associated with a marked drop in breastfeeding rates, despite the researchers reporting that breastfeeding was actively encouraged.[7] Did this happen because parents were planning to stop breastfeeding anyway? Or was it because it became increasingly difficult to maintain breastfeeding or a breast milk supply without continuation of night feeds?

The bottom line is that an infant's ability to go without a night feed is probably developmentally related, as studies have found that infants who *spontaneously* sleep for longer stretches at night without a feed (i.e. no sleep training or delaying feeds) from a very early age tend to show sleep stability at later ages as well.

Secondly, are night feeds after six months more about comfort than hunger? (And is this a bad thing?)

This may seem like a moot point, but feeding in the night is not just about hunger.[8] Some people seem to think that feeding that is unrelated to hunger is less of a valid reason to wake, and therefore worthy of elimination.

I hear a lot about people suggesting that waking to feed for comfort, rather than 'true hunger', is not a valid need. I wonder if this is rooted in our cultural tendency to perceive adult comfort-eating as linked with obesity and over-indulgence? Eating *is* a pleasurable activity – even for adults. I don't know about you, but one of my favourite things to do (though it doesn't happen very often) is to go out for a very long and decadent meal with my husband, family or friends. Eating is a social event – involving talking, laughter, and sensory stimulation. When we eat we appreciate and take pleasure in the way the food looks, smells, feels and tastes. We enjoy the surroundings and we have a chance to sit down and stop for a moment. Of course, we eat when we are hungry, but we do not overlook or consider as unnecessary the other positive aspects of eating. There are times when I am very busy and dealing with being hungry could almost be thought of as a 'task' – I eat on the run, I choose foods that are quick and will take away my hunger promptly, so I can get back to what I was doing before. Hunger and eating are therefore sometimes an *inconvenience*. But I would not say that this is the norm.

Many parents who contact me are able to discern some differences between feeds that seem to be primarily hunger-driven, and feeds that seem to be for comfort. Anecdotally, the comfort feeds are often very short, with some parents reporting that their child suckles at the breast for only a few seconds before falling asleep again. Or they offer a bottle and the child drinks only a minimal amount. These behaviours are sometimes felt to be associated with poor nighttime sleep consolidation.

I also believe, both from some research into this area, and also from listening to hundreds of parents talking about this, that sometimes a baby is fed back to sleep in the night because it *works*. What I mean is that the feed was initiated by the parent, rather than cued-for or verbally requested by the child. Many parents describe feeding back to sleep as their 'superpower', or 'trump card'. It is reliable, easy, quick and gets everyone the most amount of sleep. This is perhaps why breastfed babies are fed to sleep more, and fed in the night more, than bottle-fed babies. Literature studies do not demonstrate that bottle-fed babies wake less in the night, but they do demonstrate that breastfed babies are fed more in the night. I suspect the 'trump card factor' is at work in this phenomenon. Is this perhaps a parent-driven convenience feed, rather than an infant-driven comfort feed?

I don't have a ton of evidence I can share with you about these real-world problems. My take is a pragmatic one. I tend to suggest that if comfort feeding is beginning to get to you, then we can address it. If it isn't bothering you – leave it alone. I'll share some ideas for how to reduce or eliminate night feeds in the next chapter.

Thirdly, does night feeding (for any reason) actively promote night waking?

This is probably the hardest question to answer in a meaningful way. The reason it is so difficult is that there are so many factors to consider. The premise is that either night feeding becomes a reward that is worth waking up for, or that it somehow triggers night waking through a cascade of hormonal processes associated with appetite and satiety (the feeling of fullness and contentment after eating). Let's explore this, since it is a prevalent idea.

First of all, can feeding be thought of as a reward for an undesirable behaviour such as waking up? Well, the first thing that probably occurs to you is that waking up is normal, rather than a habit that needs to be 'broken'. But this is a grey area. Speak to any parent who is feeding their older baby back to sleep every single hour and they will almost certainly report that their child will not settle in any other way than through feeding (whether breast or bottle). It seems that while waking up in the night is normal, and night feeding is normal, the maturation of these processes towards independence progresses at different rates. Certainly, we can all develop habits that we begin to expect, or associate with certain sequences. It is not unreasonable to believe that feeding could become something that children expect to receive in order to fall asleep again. But does it therefore follow that stopping the night feeds will reduce night waking? Or will the night waking continue regardless, and you'll just have to find another way of comforting your child?

I talk to a lot of people about the need to separate responsive parenting from feeding. Feeding is just one tool with which to be responsive. You do not have to feed a child every single time they wake in order to be responsive. But you do need to do *something*. Are there other ways to be responsive that do not involve feeding, which may open up the way for other people to be involved with sleep? Probably. This is where we need to look at the whole picture of night waking in context with the age and developmental stage of your child. Given that 70 percent of children aged 6–18 months are waking for at least one night feed, it seems reasonable to use this as a baseline. If your eight-month-old baby is waking up 2–3 times in the night, then this is almost certainly reasonable. If your 10-month-old baby is waking every hour all night, then it is not

> " The hormonal control of appetite is closely balanced between the need to remain alert to eat, and the need to protect sleep through suppression of appetite. "

unreasonable to reduce this a little if it is becoming unsustainable for you.

So how does the age of your child affect the way we think about feeding to sleep? Most people don't have an issue with very young babies falling asleep feeding and feeding back to sleep in the night. It seems to be babies over the age of about 3–6 months that get people twitching. Feeding to sleep actually promotes sleep! During feeding, a baby will become calm and settled, and they have a number of complex hormones which trigger feelings of fullness, satiety, and sleep.[8-10] But what are the hormones that trigger sleep, and how do they work? This is complex stuff, but there are three hormones that are well known for their influence on appetite and sleep induction:

- Leptin: released during/after feeding or eating and decreases appetite, and increases satiety
- Cholecystokinin: decreases appetite and induces deep sleep
- Brain-derived neurotrophic factor: reduces appetite and induces sleep

So these hormones are released in response to feeding/eating and trigger a sensation of calmness and sleepiness.

Other hormones are involved with triggering appetite and wakefulness:

- Ghrelin: released by the stomach in response to emptiness. As the stomach fills, appetite falls. Makes sense!
- Orexin: promotes wakefulness and increases appetite

These hormones are triggered by stomach emptiness[11] or low blood sugar.[12,13] The slightly complex part is that it seems that just the act of being awake can also trigger appetite – so this can become a 'chicken and egg' situation. Essentially, it is possible that some babies are hungry because they are awake, rather than being awake because they are hungry. You may need to read that sentence twice! It actually makes total sense that if your body recognises that you are awake, you may need more calories, since the metabolic rate is increased during wakefulness. In other words, during wakefulness, appetite increase is an adaptation to provide the calories required to sustain alertness. There is a well-documented association between short sleep duration and increased appetite – caused by our two major appetite hormones – ghrelin (which increases) and leptin (which decreases). The overall effect is to make you hungrier and less satisfied. However, the studies that have explored these links are done with adults, so again we simply don't know if they can be applied to children and infants. Fundamentally, the hormonal control of appetite is closely balanced between the need to remain alert to eat, and the need to protect sleep through suppression of appetite.

At what point this tightly maintained balance gets triggered is hard to say, as the studies that examine these hormones have not explored their effects in infants. Therefore, any suggestion about the relevance of this in infancy is speculative. I tend, therefore, to be guided by what is manageable and sustainable for families in the light of their child's age.

One recent sleep intervention programme actively encourages feeding to sleep, because of these well-known biological sleep drivers. They argue that if an infant becomes sleepy during a feed, and then is abruptly woken to avoid them falling asleep feeding, they may associate feeling sleepy with sudden wakefulness. They also point out that feeding to sleep is easy, quick and reliable, and keeping a baby awake during and after feeding is difficult and unreliable – so the whole process can increase stress, reduce parental confidence and cause an infant's feed-sleep-wake cycle to become disrupted.[14] It is refreshing to hear an alternative approach to sleep that does not make parents feel like they are 'getting it all wrong'. Whether this applies to all babies, or just certain ages or temperaments, remains to be seen, but it is certainly worth thinking about if you notice that your baby always seems really sleepy after feeding, and then startles and gets upset when you try to put them down to sleep 'drowsy but awake'. If this happens, you may want to abandon the strategy for a while and relax a little about sleepy feeds.

On a practical level, with very young babies it is almost impossible to stop them falling asleep feeding. Part of the reason for this is that they are unable to sustain long bouts of wakefulness. If you think about it, by the time you have realised your baby is cueing to be fed, and you have changed them, then either breast or bottle-fed them, burped them and dealt with any nappy explosions, it may well be time to sleep again. For some babies, the short amount of awake time they can tolerate between feeds means that they are almost guaranteed to fall asleep feeding. This will persist until their tolerable awake window lengthens enough for them to be able to sustain some awake time after a feed.

The astute among you may be wondering about the effects of appetite on circadian rhythm. Again, there is almost no research in this area, and the research that does exist tends to relate to adults, and sleep pathology, rather than normal infants. For example, adults with night eating syndrome have a delay in their circadian appetite control despite normal sleep-wake rhythm.[15] But this is a sleep pathology, whereas infants who feed at night are normal. How relevant is this to babies? Another example is jet lag and the impacts on appetite and sleep. We know that it can take a few days for your body to adjust to a different time zone. Is it possible that babies or children can adjust their circadian-linked appetite timings by habitually eating or feeding at certain times? Again, this is a hugely complex and grey area, because night feeds are biologically normal and necessary in a young infant. At what point might their circadian rhythm be a factor in appetite regulation? It is certainly true that there is an inter-relationship between circadian rhythm, appetite and metabolism.[16] Another study[17] found that circadian rhythm is affected by food timing. This study found that the body clock is affected by significantly different meal times. It effectively shifts the circadian rhythm. But the meal times were shifted by five hours. What about smaller variations?

Finally, does night feeding affect daytime appetite?

On the face of it, this sounds like a sensible mechanism – if you stuff yourself at night, you'll eat less in the day. It is certainly possible to shift your circadian rhythm timings through appetite modification and timing of food intake.[18] However, this would usually require other environmental cues, such as light and social activity, as well. In fact, the research studies we have on sleep deprivation and appetite would suggest the opposite – that if you're sleep deprived, you will tend to eat more.[19] Another study found that less sleep is associated with higher food intake in 8–11 year-olds.[20] It is hard to find scientific papers that corroborate the notion that feeding in the night disrupts eating in the day. There is a wealth of literature demonstrating the opposite – but these studies tend to be in school-age children, and are addressing the issue from a childhood obesity point of view.

Anecdotally, many people report that if their child feeds frequently at night they tend not to want breakfast. Yet it is also a common observance that children are often grazers in the day anyway. They may just not be a big fan of breakfast! So, once again, this could be chicken and egg – is the child feeding all night because they have a 'grazing' pattern of eating which is mirrored in the daytime? Or are they feeding all night because they don't eat well in the day? Or is it a vicious circle of feeding all night, reducing daytime appetite? Is night feeding a safety net – providing important calories and nutrition to a child with low appetite? Does it depend on whether the night feeds are substantial or momentary?

I would suggest that you look at your child's eating patterns in general. Do they eat well in the day apart from breakfast? Do they actually graze all day irrespective of feeding? For example:

Maya has been told that her one-year-old daughter Josie does not eat solids well because she is up all night feeding. Maya tried to limit feeds in the night in the hope that Josie would eat well the next day. Josie was still thoroughly uninterested in breakfast, and her appetite for the rest of the day remained unchanged. Maya concluded that night feeding was having no impact on Josie's daytime eating patterns, and considering that her weight was normal, and Josie was healthy and thriving, decided to just let the night feeds run their course.

On the other hand:

Brian and Claire were convinced that their 11-month-old son was stuck in a rut of having large feeds in the night, and essentially 'sleeping through' the day. Noah would wake up at least every 2-3 hours and have a really substantial feed. Claire described breast fullness and Noah guzzling milk from both breasts, then seeming content to go for long periods in the daytime without anything at all. Claire noted that the behaviour started when Noah began to be more interested in his surroundings at about four months, and he would regularly last for 8-9 hours in the daytime without any breastfeeds, then compensate at night. Claire decided to gently hold her son and not feed him after 3am one day as an experiment, to see if he would then eat breakfast and breastfeed in the morning. She noticed that Noah was much more interested in breakfast the next morning.

I cannot tell you which way this is likely to play out in your situation. I truly think that for some children, grazing all day and night is their feeding pattern, whereas for others, like Noah, it may be that your little one has 'reverse cycled' their feeding pattern. You may need to experiment, keep an open mind, and be prepared to be flexible.

Night feeds and milk supply

Let's think a little more about the association between night feeding and milk supply. A milk supply that is still becoming established may suffer from long breaks between feeds. Long gaps are usually not a great idea for young babies, for safety, weight, and their energy and caloric needs, as well as maternal milk supply. But will a milk supply and baby be compromised by having limits placed on night feeds at eight months, or 10 months? It is almost certainly not necessary to feed every 1-2 hours with an older baby in terms of their nutritional requirements or to maintain milk production. But where is the line? What other factors do we need to consider? Does age matter – and if so, at what age can limits be placed on night feeds safely?

At six months, milk supply is generally well-established, so in theory allowing longer breaks between feeds is unlikely to impact milk production overall. However, it does depend on individual factors, including a mother's comfort level when her breasts become fuller, and storage capacity. Essentially, one mother's breast may be able to hold a maximum of 50ml of milk, while another breast may be able to store 250ml. The storage capacity will greatly influence the frequency of feeding of an infant. If a mother has a small milk storage capacity, her milk supply and her infant's weight may only be maintained by frequent feeds. On the other hand, there may be more room for manoeuvre if the mother has a larger storage capacity – assuming of course that her infant is able to drink a larger volume in one feeding session. Variables like these would not necessarily be known (or even cared about) in advance by a mother who was feeding responsively, but may become apparent and problematic if night feeds are spaced out or eliminated.

I suggest an individualised approach to decision-making about night feed spacing. If your baby is thriving, experiment with a small increase in feeding interval to see what impact this has on your comfort level and milk supply. If there is no obvious negative impact, you may want to increase the interval further. If you become uncomfortably full or your milk supply dips, then you may want to get some support from a breastfeeding counsellor or IBCLC.

Night feeds and fertility

I come across a substantial number of parents who want to stop night feeds to try to get their fertility to return so that they can have another child. Every woman has a different level of sensitivity to hormones. For some people, their period returns while they are fully breastfeeding – day and night. For others, it comes back when their little one is no longer exclusively breastfeeding: either their little one is having some formula, or solids. Still others find that breastfeeding has to reduce quite substantially – often overnight – for the return of their period, and for another group of women fertility does not return until they completely stop breastfeeding. The lactational amenorrhea method is known to be a fairly good method of contraception, but there is significant variability between individuals. An example:

Grace called for sleep support when her daughter Tori was 10 months old. Grace had no issue with Tori's night waking habits. Tori woke about 3–4 times in the night and Grace was happy to bed-share and feed her back to sleep. However, Grace was 42 years old, and it had taken over three years to conceive Tori. Since her period had not yet returned, she wanted to explore the possibility of reducing or even eliminating night feeds in order for her fertility to return. She was mindful of her age, and did not want to risk waiting too long.

Bear in mind that if your primary reason for wanting to stop night feeds is the return of your fertility, this is by no means an exact science. If your fertility has already returned, you do not need to stop breastfeeding or night feeding for the sake of your unborn baby (unless you want to). The other thing to bear in mind is that you may feel quite conflicted or even have feelings of guilt attached to this decision – it's an emotive process. Please get support with this from a breastfeeding counsellor or IBCLC who has experience dealing with this compassionately. One final word of warning: your fertility may have returned by stealth. A lot of women find that their period does not come back because they are already pregnant – rule that out before you embark on night weaning!

What about night feeds for formula-fed babies?

Is it a different story for formula fed babies? Or babies fed expressed breastmilk in the night? Is it easier to organise the day so that your child has more of their daily caloric needs met during the daytime? The short answer is that it may be possible to orchestrate feedings so that they are clustered during your waking hours. However, there is no evidence that this will reduce night waking. Most of the previous sections will still apply if your baby is bottle-fed - the only part that will be irrelevant is the section discussing the impact of long gaps between feeds on milk production. Sometimes parents combination feed - a mixture of formula and breast milk - either from the breast or bottle. There is no evidence to suggest that breastfed, formula-fed or combination-fed babies sleep vastly differently from each other, especially after the first 3-4 months. The main difference with bottle-feeding a baby is that you'll need to make sure you keep a vague idea of how much milk your little one is drinking in 24 hours. If you feed them literally every time they wake up there is a risk they will be overfed - which I'm sure you know already. You'll need to find other ways of helping your baby back to sleep when they wake in the night.

What about falling asleep feeding?

Feeding to sleep is one practice I am fairly certain you have heard about, and perhaps you have even given some thought to it. Does your baby fall asleep feeding? Have you been told to stop doing this to improve sleep? Have you tried it? One of the big ideas in sleep research is that of allowing your baby to fall asleep on their own. And many studies have found that not feeding to sleep is associated with better nighttime sleep.[21-26] This makes sense on one level - if a baby feels safe and calm and gets into the habit of going to sleep without any help, then this could perpetuate the practice. A key message in most sleep guidelines or sleep studies is that an infant's ability to fall asleep without a parent's assistance is a key predictor of sleeping through the night. One very large study (over 10,000 babies) found that breastfeeding back to sleep was associated with more night waking and less consolidated sleep. In fact, they did not find any difference in the number of nighttime awakenings between breast and formula-fed babies, but noticed that the breastfed babies were more likely to be nursed back to sleep - which seemed to be independently related to more fragmented sleep.[27]

In the middle of the night, when parents are tired, I believe what often happens is that a baby or toddler wakes for comfort, and does not specifically require a feed. What they do require is responsiveness – but this responsiveness does not *have* to involve feeding. But sometimes a feed is offered as a quick way of getting a baby back to sleep. The 'trump card' sleep tool when all other strategies fail. I vividly remember my husband asking me what our youngest needed after I'd come through from resettling her for the fourth time in three hours one evening many years ago. He asked me: 'Did she need a feed?'. It's a simple enough question, but it got me thinking. My response was: 'I don't know if a feed was what she needed, but a feed was what she got'. In other words, I played the feed trump card a lot. Can babies become accustomed to the trump card? Yes, I think they probably can. If this is what *always* happens, night after night, it is not hard to imagine that babies will come to expect that this is just the way they fall back to sleep again. They don't mean to make you tired. It doesn't occur to them that this might be inconvenient.

It can get confusing though, because are the babies who feed frequently in the night for parental convenience or out of desperation for sleep, to be treated differently from the babies who fall asleep feeding? Another large study did not find a clinical difference in sleep outcome between the babies who were put to sleep awake, versus the babies who fell asleep in arms or feeding.[28] Given that it can take quite a lot of hard work and consistency over time to put a baby to bed awake, if it doesn't work this is a real waste of time and effort.

Is perhaps feeding to sleep a different issue from feeding *back* to sleep in the night? Do we need to separate the times when babies could potentially be comforted in other ways than feeding, from the times when babies wake up genuinely hungry (as is normal for 6–18 month olds)? It is much more convenient and easier to remember if we have one rule for everything, everyone and every time – such as 'never feed your baby to sleep'. But what if this isn't true? I have met hundreds of children and infants who can feed to sleep at bedtime and not wake excessively in the night. Did they get lucky? Or is there something about modifying the parental response in the night so that we always offer comfort, but don't always offer a feed? Of course, the great advantage to many exhausted breastfeeding mothers is that if comfort can be reliably offered in other ways, then it opens up the opportunity for *someone else* to help in the night.

Academic stalemate?

My observation is that articles, books, sleep practitioners and researchers who suggest that night feeding and feeding to sleep are associated with sleep problems are trying to *prioritise sleep*. Articles, books, lactation professionals and researchers who suggest that night feeding is normal, common and protective are trying to *prioritise breastfeeding and responsive bottle-feeding*. Does it follow that either group is right or wrong? Or are we just coming at this from two different angles? With a foot firmly in both camps, I can genuinely see both perspectives. One possible take is that while night feeding and feeding to sleep (whether by breast or bottle) are entirely normal, they are also incontrovertibly associated with more night waking. Reducing feeding at night or supporting babies and children to fall asleep without feeding may improve sleep, but it is not spontaneously normal behaviour for a lot of children. There are also other factors, such as temperament, individual feeding variability, health and many others which may affect feeding and sleeping behaviours independently.

It is possible that modifying normal infant behaviour may improve sleep consolidation, but we are now talking about a deviation from the norm. Whenever we are talking about deviating from the norm, we have to accept that firstly there may be consequences of doing this, and secondly that this is not easy.

Alongside the theoretical information we have available, we also need to acknowledge the human factor. Night waking is hard, and there are strategies available to parents (albeit not always well known) that can potentially improve sleep to the point where it becomes manageable. There seems to be a willingness to consider a middle ground from professionals who advocate for gentle parenting and responsive feeding that understands that infant-parent sleep can sometimes be very difficult and may respond to simple, respectful sleep strategies.[29]

Hopefully by now you've established that the link between feeding and sleep is perhaps not as straightforward as it seems. Here is a summary, just in case you've jumped to this section:

- Children wake up in the night for many reasons – feeding is just one of them
- Feeding to sleep is sometimes related to hunger, but sometimes also

for infant-led comfort, or parent-led convenience – the sleep 'trump card'

- Most babies aged 6-18 months wake in the night 1-3 times, and most of them have at least one night feed
- Feeding to sleep often promotes sleep
- Wakefulness increases appetite
- Preventing babies from falling asleep feeding may potentially upset their sleep-wake pattern, if they are startled awake just as they fall asleep
- Stopping night feeds does not always stop night waking
- Night feeding may have an element of circadian rhythmicity, but it is likely to be multi-factorial
- Daytime appetite may not be affected by nighttime feeding in some children
- It is possible that children get into the habit of feeding back to sleep and come to prefer this over other ways of receiving comfort
- Reducing night feeds may have a negative impact on breastfeeding duration in some parents – depending on infant age, feeding behaviour, storage capacity, infant appetite and milk supply
- Formula-fed babies are just as likely to wake in the night, but are less likely to be fed back to sleep
- Falling asleep feeding is normal, common and complex to unpick
- Responsive feeding and responsive parenting are not always the same thing. It is okay to offer a child other ways to receive comfort and reassurance if feeding to sleep has become excessive or unsustainable

How do you gently reduce night feeds?

If your little one is feeding very frequently in the night – more than every two hours over the age of six months, or if it is becoming unmanageable – then you could try to reduce the feeds. Please bear the following in mind:

- Consider whether your child has an underlying feeding problem that would be better resolved with specialist feeding input
- Does your child have a medical problem that is the root cause of their frequent feeding and/or discomfort?

- Are you wanting to stop night feeds because they are unmanageable, or is it due to social pressure, unwanted advice or because you feel that you are the only one still feeding your child in the night?
- Is your only reason for reducing or stopping night feeds the promise of more sleep? If so, then this is not a guaranteed strategy to improve sleep

If you are sure that reducing or stopping night feeds is the right choice for you and your family, then there are many ways of going about this. I'll list them in order of ease of implementation, with the easiest first.

1. Gradually increasing the length of time between feeds

Gradually lengthening the gap between feeds by adding in additional caregiving activity to delay the feed seemed to be an effective strategy in breastfed infants in one study, though it would depend on the maternal milk supply being able to cope with a gradual increase in time between feeds.[30] It would work just as well for a bottle-fed baby. Essentially, you could add in delay tactics, so that before you know it, you have delayed perhaps half an hour by cuddling, nappy changing, or holding. Most of the time, this involves no crying at all.

2. Placing some limits on night feeds

This is a little more directive as a strategy. It works well for some parents who want to have a more concrete idea of what to expect, and allows other people to help settle the child. There's nothing very complex about this. Instead of feeding every time your child wakes up, you might decide on a reasonable limit. For example, if your little one tends to wake every 40 minutes, you might initially say 'no feeds until 9pm', having fed them at 7pm. You don't need to make a big jump. I would usually recommend doing this in very small increments. Going from hourly to two-hourly feeds makes a big difference to some people! Once this is working well, you might extend the limit and say 'no feeds until 10pm', or whatever. Go at your child's pace, and if you're breastfeeding, this allows you to keep an eye on how your milk supply and breast comfort is coping as well.

3. Reducing the length of the feed

This is quite an arbitrary way of reducing night feeds, but it appeals to some people. It works especially well for babies who are drinking large volumes from the breast in the night. Milk of course does not flow at a constant rate, but reducing the length of feed will eventually reduce the feed to a momentary one. Let's say you decide your arbitrary maximum feed length is 10 minutes (you may initially set it longer if your little one takes a long time to feed). You would initially feed for 10 minutes, then take your little one off and hold them close, offering them a cuddle, kisses, stroking and gentle verbal reassurance. They may settle quickly in your arms – you never know! Reduce the feed by 30 seconds, or a minute, every few days – be led by your baby and go at the pace that feels right for you, your little one, and your breast comfort.

4. Reducing the volume of feed

For babies who are bottle-fed with formula or expressed milk, you could try to reduce the volume – this is essentially the same idea as point 3, but with amounts rather than time. Reduce the volume by a small amount every few days until the feed is very minimal. Then try to drop it, perhaps shifting the feeds before and after it.

5. Disassociating feeding from falling asleep

This is based on the idea that you want your baby or child to find other ways of falling asleep, but you appreciate that night feeds are normal at their age. The problem with feeding your baby at some wake-ups, and offering other forms of comfort in between, is that for some babies this seems to be confusing. While some babies can tolerate some inconsistency, it seems that some like to know where they stand and do better with a single consistent approach. This is hard if the night feeds are entirely appropriate at your child's age. One way of getting around this is to always settle them without a feed, so that they get a clear and consistent message, but offer them a sleepy feed or dreamfeed to meet their needs for feeding in the night. People have lots of opinions about dreamfeeds. Some people suggest that they may disrupt feed-sleep-wake patterns because infants are being fed when they haven't cued to feed, and you may be waking them when they are deeply asleep. On the other hand, it may help to stop a wake-up that is triggered by hunger, allowing you to consistently get your baby back to sleep, or set limits on feeds while maintaining your settling approach in the night without feeding. The truth is that they seem to work brilliantly for some babies, and are completely unhelpful for others. I'll leave you to make up your own mind.

6. Stopping feeds altogether

This may sound hardcore – but in certain circumstances it may be entirely the right thing to do. I almost always recommend and advocate for a slower and more gradual reduction in night feeds, but there are two main times when stopping them completely may be appropriate. They are: extreme parental circumstances, and very momentary but very frequent feeds in a persistent older toddler.

If you or your partner have become unwell, you need to start treatment that is contraindicated in breastfeeding, or you have a sudden crisis that makes night feeding very difficult or impossible, then sometimes abrupt night weaning is the only thing you can do. You will need to support your little one extensively, and you may find it easier to involve your partner. For older toddlers who are on and off the breast, sometimes placing limits can almost feel like a 'tease' – giving them something they want briefly, and then removing it. Sometimes it is easier, and ultimately kinder, depending on your child's personality, to night wean completely with kindness and compassion.

Night feeding is probably one of the most controversial areas after crying it out. Maybe you're surprised at the lack of hard evidence. Maybe you're not surprised in the least. But at least you know, and you can make an informed choice.

The tired parent's summary

- Night feeding and night waking are separate but related issues.
- Stopping night feeds is often thought to be the key to stopping night waking. In reality, it's only one part of the story.
- Despite plenty of people saying that night feeds after six months are unnecessary, there is actually very little evidence that this is a universally realistic expectation.
- Night feeds are not just about hunger and caloric need.
- Night feeds actually promote sleep, so removing them can sometimes worsen sleep.
- Night feeding and daytime appetite are inter-linked, but more complex and variable than many people believe.
- There is very little evidence that formula-fed babies wake up less often than breastfed babies. Even if they feed less, the waking patterns are usually very similar.

- Babies probably can and do develop a preference for feeding back to sleep. Some parents don't have a problem with this, while others find it frustrating.
- Reducing or stopping night feeds is sometimes desired or required by parents and this can be achieved gently and respectfully, without leaving babies to cry alone.

Chapter nine

Why not leave them to cry?

→ Welcome to the controversial question of whether leaving children to cry is a good idea or not. Is it merely loud, slightly harrowing for parents, but ultimately short-lived and effective at solving sleep disruption? Or is it stressful, potentially affecting parent-child trust and attachment and having no guarantee of success? Crying strategies are known by many terms, including:

- Extinction – also known as cry-it-out
- Modified/graduated extinction – also known as controlled crying
- Controlled comforting
- Spaced soothing
- Rapid return
- Crying down

There are a bewildering number of books, studies and blogs claiming to give you the answers. Many recent books continue to say that cry-it-out is not harmful.[1,2] Even public guidelines for children's community services endorse crying it out.[3] The truth is, whatever it is you want to hear, you will probably be able to find a paper to back you up. But what is the actual evidence? Is there enough evidence either way? Are there complexities that haven't been studied? Are all children affected in the same way? And how does all this fit with how you want to parent?

Let's try to unpick this thorny issue, and as I do so, I am mindful that this is a highly contentious and emotive debate. It is never my intention to be sanctimonious. After all, most people a) trust the research that they read, and b) are just doing the best they can, with the information available at the time.

What is the central argument about?

Essentially, the debate revolves around whether leaving children to cry alone causes harm. When children are left alone, have an unmet need, or experience a negative emotion that they are incapable of processing, they mount a stress response. A stress response is normal – we must be able to react quickly to threats or dangers. No problem so far. But is there a potential problem with prolonged, repeated stress? If there is, what are the potential harms, and does it depend on the child's age? The length of time they are left to cry? How many days it takes for the child to start to sleep? Does it always work? On the flip side, what about the reported negative impacts of prolonged sleep deprivation on parents – relationship difficulties, increase in postnatal depression and trouble with daily functioning? Does long-term fatigue impact a parent's ability to sensitively respond to their child? In other words, does the potential risk of leaving a child to cry outweigh the potential impacts of sleep deprivation?

When leaving children or babies to cry, the theory is that they learn to fall asleep independently. Some people use it to deal with an established sleep 'problem' – such as their child only falling asleep with a particular trigger. The theory is that continuation of the previous sleep trigger serves to reinforce the behaviour, and parental presence or the trigger becomes a 'reward'. In this case, the child will cry to protest the absence of the trigger. With a continued non-response, the child eventually falls asleep. Proponents of the technique argue that the child has 'learned' to fall asleep independently. There is some debate over whether they have in fact learned anything at all, besides just accepting that nobody will come. Other people use this technique to teach children to fall asleep independently before any habit can become established. This is common in families where parents return to work after a short parental leave and the pressure for a child to be sleeping through the night is high. Sometimes the technique is practised on babies as young as six weeks old, though most researchers do not suggest it before six months.

What do studies in favour of controlled crying/cry-it-out claim?

Plenty of studies claim that there is no harm in leaving babies to cry.[4] Some studies suggest that low parental tolerance to crying is one factor associated with sleep problems.[5] Mostly, research questions present the idea that babies and children should be able to sleep for long stretches, without needing parental assistance, and that this independence in sleep predicts long-term positive sleep outcomes. The age at which infants 'should' be sleeping through the night is slightly variable across studies, but the vast majority claim that night feeds are no longer necessary after six months. Some studies suggest that sleep training can commence while babies still need night feeds, and that training them to fall asleep independently, without feeding or needing to be held to sleep, means that they will be less likely to experience sleep difficulties later on.

There have been three main studies in recent years.[6-8] They have all concluded that controlled crying or cry-it-out is effective at improving sleep, reduces the likelihood of postnatal depression and has no negative consequences on infant mental health or attachment.

The first study[9] included 328 mother-baby pairs. The families were recruited in Australia when the infants were seven months old and were randomised into two groups. They either received sleep education or underwent a graduated-extinction program. The study found that fewer mothers in the graduated-extinction group had postnatal depression when their child was two years old than the control group. However, there was *limited improvement in sleep outcome* for both the control group and the intervention group.

This study did not really say anything about the safety of sleep training. It mainly reported a small but statistically significant reduction in the rate of postnatal depression. You might expect to see this effect anyway. There is a phenomenon known as the Hawthorn effect, when participants report a difference just by virtue of being in a research study. As well as this, the participants were seen by a psychologist – which is likely to have had an impact on their mental health. Sometimes just knowing that you are doing *something* constructive is enough to make someone feel better – essentially a placebo effect. But the main news with this study is that it did not find that either strategy significantly helped improve sleep.

The second study[10] was actually a follow-up of the earlier Hiscock study and aimed to prove that there was no long-term harm caused by graduated extinction (controlled crying). The same 328 mother-baby pairs who took part in the original study were contacted and assessed at the age of six. Salivary cortisol samples were taken when the children were six years old, and the study reported that the cortisol levels were similar in the intervention and control groups – although the actual data is not provided.

We firstly have to remember that the original study did not conclude that either the sleep education or the graduated extinction significantly helped improve sleep. As well as this, there were a number of errors with this study which make interpretation and recommendations for practice very difficult. The study lost nearly half their sample to follow-up, and not only this, but the 46 percent of children lost to follow-up were largely those who had been identified as high-risk. So arguably those most at risk of a long-term negative effect were not reassessed. The main error with this study is that a cortisol sample was only taken six years after the original intervention. No sample was taken before the intervention, during, immediately after, or at any time point other than six years post-intervention. This is a big problem, because normal cortisol levels change over time. Without knowing what the children's original cortisol level was, we cannot actually make any sensible interpretation of this study.

The third and most recent study[11] recruited 43 babies aged between six and 16 months. This study aimed to find out whether graduated extinction, an intervention called fading or supportive care had any effect on sleep, maternal and infant stress, and long-term parent-infant attachment and behaviour. Cortisol samples were taken from the babies before the treatment, and at three points after the treatment, and mothers' stress levels were also measured before and after treatment as well. The Strange Situation test was used after treatment to assess attachment.

Firstly, this was a very small study. It found that in the graduated-extinction group, 46 percent of the children were insecurely attached. In the control group, 39 percent of the children were insecurely attached. The population prevalence of insecure attachment is about 30 percent. The problem here is that this is not a representative sample of the population. Were the children experiencing sleep problems *because* they were insecure? Or could the insecure attachment be due to the intervention? Was sleep problematic because of *other* factors to start with, such as stressful home environment, lack of emotional availability and so on? Could the presence of sleep problems due to underlying factors have led these parents to pursue a sleep intervention? Both groups showed a high proportion of insecure infants, but the level was higher in the graduated-extinction group. Furthermore, the Strange Situation test should be used on children aged 12 to 20 months, and is not necessarily a reliable way of measuring attachment outside of this age range.[13] In this study, the oldest children were 16 months at the onset of the treatment, and therefore would have been 28 months at follow-up, which is well outside of the age range for this test. Finally, cortisol samples were taken before and after the intervention – however, the reference cortisol value would have dropped in that time anyway, due to the natural drop in cortisol after one year. So, compared to the baseline, the cortisol value several months later is almost meaningless.

What about studies claiming that controlled crying is bad for babies?

The opposing argument is that babies cannot regulate their emotional state, so if they become stressed, they lack the ability to be able to self-regulate. One study of four-month-old infants found that even after sleep onset, the cortisol levels of the infants who had been left to cry remained elevated – indicating that the infants still had an activated stress response.[13] The study has been criticised because unmodified extinction (cry-it-out) is generally not recommended until six months, and further, the infants were in a clinical sleep setting, which could have falsely elevated their stress levels. As well as this, we have no follow-up cortisol samples to assess whether the babies eventually calmed down and how long that process took. However, the study is concerning, and we have no evidence at the present time to reassure us about when cortisol levels return to baseline after an intervention such as controlled crying or cry-it-out. Other studies suggest that even if there are initial improvements in sleep, the effect is not always sustained, and the intervention needs to be repeated.[14]

The impact of sensitive parenting and attachment on stress and sleep

There is actually quite a lot of research to suggest that early, responsive, sensitive care from a parent who is emotionally available, and shows high warmth (cuddles, kisses, praise, encouragement) promotes optimal development of the stress response system.[15]

In fact, there is a substantial amount of research that tells us that promoting secure attachment may improve sleep.[16-19] These research studies consistently find that there is an association between insecurely attached children and long-term, disrupted sleep. I'm mindful as I write this that if your child does not sleep well, you may now suddenly panic that your child is insecure! That is absolutely not what I am saying. For what it's worth, my children are securely attached and have both been fragmented and short sleepers. Just because your child does not sleep a solid stretch, does not mean they are insecure – after all, there are many factors. What it does mean, is that both secure and insecurely attached children can have disrupted sleep, but insecurely attached children *more often* sleep in a fragmented pattern. Optimising attachment is therefore a good idea, but it does not guarantee your child will sleep.

How does nurturing and responsive care affect stress?

Well, at the risk of sounding like I am obsessed, we need to go back to our friend cortisol again. Hormones are amazing little substances and often have clever complexes, negative feedback loops and adaptive processes that make them work in the most efficient way possible. Cortisol is no different.

Our cells need to be primed to respond to cortisol. One of the ways we can do this is through glucocorticoid receptors (GRs) that attach themselves to cortisol. This allows the activated GR complex to enter a cell and interact with it, including its DNA. This might sound like some kind of alien stress invasion, but GRs are the good guys. They enable us to respond *efficiently* to stress. The more GRs we have, the more sensitive we are to cortisol – meaning we need to release less cortisol to have an effective stress response. It also means we can recover faster from stress. If we have fewer GRs, we need more cortisol to have the same effective stress response, and we also have a slower recovery from stress.

Your stress response has lots of clever feedback loops. When you are stressed or threatened, your brain sends a signal in the form of a chemical messenger – corticotropin releasing hormone (CRH) – which causes more cortisol to be made in your adrenal glands. But the really smart bit is that your brain also detects the rising cortisol. It's very like a thermostat. If your home is too hot, the thermostat sends a message to your boiler to turn off. The heat drops, and if it drops below a certain level, the boiler kicks back in again – but the whole process is permanently monitored by the thermostat. Your brain is like the thermostat – when it detects rising cortisol, it sends a message to your adrenal glands (boiler) to stop releasing cortisol. So, this is supposed to be an efficient system – allowing us to respond quickly to a danger, and then calm down again afterwards. An exaggerated stress response leads to a weakened immune system – not a great idea. So chronic stress can raise our baseline cortisol, though it is unclear how long this process takes to become upregulated, or if it can recover.

Back to those little GRs. More GRs cause your brain to make less CRH. This means you will release less cortisol. Your stress response is more efficient, and you have a faster recovery from stress. People with chronic stress have a cortisol level that is permanently elevated. The really amazing thing is that it appears that close, nurturing, responsive care in infancy is linked with an upregulation of an epigenetic process that causes more GRs to be produced. Remember more GRs equals less CRH equals less cortisol required, which means a more efficient stress response and faster stress recovery. The genetic change is stable and permanently affects our stress response.[20] In contrast, a lack of responsive care causes the gene that is responsible for making GRs to be switched off. The child will have fewer GRs, and therefore will have an elevated stress response and slower recovery from stress.[21]

The bottom line: it's a good idea to kiss, hold, cuddle, stroke and wear your baby, respond promptly and not leave them alone to cry. It seems that anything we can do to promote attachment and bonding is likely to have long-term positive benefits for your child. I'm not promising that this alone will lead to more sleep, but it's certainly the justification we need to keep doing what feels instinctive.

Which questions remain unanswered?

One of the main problems is that the studies so far have assumed that one or two cortisol samples during the day are sufficient to assess for a stress response. One study used the Strange Situation test as well, though there were some problems with using that test. However, several assumptions were made about cortisol at the outset of the studies that have been done so far. Researchers have assumed that there is a standard range of cortisol, and have not accounted for variability between age. The Gradisar study measured cortisol at three different time points, and at different times of day, but the Price study did not.

Cortisol levels rise on a month-by-month basis over the first 12 months[22] but then fall between the ages of 1-6 years.[23] As well as these long-term changes, cortisol levels also fluctuate during the day, with higher levels being reported in the morning and the lowest levels a few hours after nighttime sleep onset. As well as this, your circadian cortisol profile and your stress response are independent of each other. This makes total sense, because otherwise, if we were exposed to threat or danger at a time when our circadian cortisol level was low, we would be unable to react. That would be a serious design fault.

Cortisol values also vary between gender and between individuals with different day/night timing preferences in response to their natural circadian rhythm. So people with early-bird chronotypes will have a differently timed circadian cortisol profile to people with night-owl chronotypes.[24] This may have been a factor in the studies, as chronotype begins to shift by the toddler years towards a slightly later wake-up time.[25] Comparing people's circadian cortisol is difficult – especially with very small samples and using children of different ages. It's simply too confusing to get meaningful information.

The final problem that jumps out is that the cortisol released during stress is independent of the circadian rhythm cortisol value.[26] While people who are stressed will have a raised circadian cortisol profile, we do not know how long it takes for the cortisol value to be upregulated in this way. So if researchers assume that children who have become permanently stressed reflect this in their circadian cortisol value, we could have a problem. If the two are only associated, but not linked, then measuring a circadian cortisol value and using this to try to prove that there is no evidence of a stress response is a long shot. The Middlemiss study and the Gradisar and Price studies were therefore measuring two different cortisol values.

In the Middlemiss study, cortisol samples were taken shortly after the intervention, and the cortisol level was still elevated. In the Price and Gradisar studies, the cortisol was measured at a time when the children were not stressed. As well as this, the Middlemiss study measured cortisol values in a clinical sleep setting, while the Gradisar study measured cortisol in a home setting. What difference the environment made to the children is uncertain, but one study[27] mused that cortisol levels may be raised in an institutional setting. Therefore, the studies were measuring *different cortisol processes* in different places, with different-aged children – you cannot check a circadian cortisol level which is in the normal range and compare with a stressed sample and deduce that one study was right or wrong. They were simply measuring different values.

So cortisol-related confounders include:

- Cortisol values vary with age
- Cortisol values vary with gender
- Values may differ in different settings
- Cortisol increases initially until 12 months, and then falls until age six
- Cortisol values vary with the time of day
- The value will be different depending on chronotype
- Cortisol values have a normal range – if you do not check a baseline (as in the Price study) then you cannot tell if the value is raised from the baseline. It may still be in the normal range, and yet be elevated
- Circadian cortisol is a separate process to stress cortisol – we do not know enough yet about how the two inter-relate
- GRs affect the production of cortisol, and this seems to be set early in life. It could be that the stress response is set earlier than the studies have so far measured – if the children were already exhibiting a raised stress response, it is possible that we would not see the true effect.

The implications of this are huge when the central argument relies on cortisol levels being a reliable indicator of whether or not the infant stress response is affected by being left to cry alone. If we cannot be sure of

> ❝ The bottom line: it's a good idea to kiss, hold, cuddle, stroke and wear your baby, respond promptly and not leave them alone to cry. ❞

this, then there is no way we can recommend that leaving infants to cry is harmless. Furthermore, we have different studies measuring cortisol levels at different time points relative to the intervention, with different ages of children and differences in the exact type of intervention. The three main pro cry-it-out studies all claim to add to the burden of evidence from previous studies, yet all of them are flawed to start with.

At the present time, I genuinely believe we have insufficient evidence to conclusively prove the safety of cry-it-out or controlled crying. There is no study that has examined cry-it-out and controlled crying and accounted for all the confounding factors and variables. The study would ideally be large, cross-cultural, conducted at home, confirmed with actigraphy, with a baseline cortisol, as well as multiple cortisol measurements, with an induced stress cortisol sample to reassess for the true reflection on the stress response. Such a study would be complex and probably impossible to gain ethical approval for.

Popular books and guidelines

Many books advocate the use of cry-it-out or controlled crying. Ignoring this advice can earn you labels such as 'martyr'. It is often seen as the inevitable outcome to a difficult sleep situation. But central to this is the pathologising of normal infant behaviour. It is unhelpful that this is an ingrained part of our child-rearing culture. Because it is such an emotive argument, people have turned to science and research to try to prove their point. Only as we have seen, the studies that are cited are not as helpful as we need them to be to make an informed choice. The bizarre thing is that some extremely intelligent and eminent people have read these studies and not commented on the flaws. This makes me angry on your behalf. How are parents supposed to make a decision for their families when they don't know who to trust? It is a sad fact that people sometimes only see what they want or expect to see. The more we look for 'evidence' of something we want to see, the more we see it. It's even got a name – the 'illusory truth effect'.[28] Everyone seems to be susceptible to it. One recent book claimed to have thoroughly examined *all* the research,[29] while others claim that they will thoroughly explain why there is 'no harm in leaving your baby to cry', only to give you one paragraph citing the flawed research I have just critiqued.[30] You would hope that national guidelines would have a more unbiased and critical analysis of the available research, but apparently not.[31]

I can see the appeal of wanting to find that cry-it-out is harmless. I really can. After all, if it is quick, the instructions are simple, it is effective, and it reduces postnatal mental health problems – it's a no-brainer. The problem is, I'm really sceptical that those are the conclusions we can draw at the present time. So it seems we are at an impasse. The only thing everyone can agree on is that we all genuinely want what's best for families.

Variability of child response

A crystal ball would be useful to know which children are likely to struggle more with cry-it-out. Advocates of sleep training claim that it is quick and effective. Do I believe that *all* children are harmed by sleep training? I think that it's probably not sensible to say that. While I have personally never used it as an intervention, I have met numerous people whose child cried briefly for 5–10 minutes a few times, and then slept well thereafter. I do not think it is likely in the context of a secure environment, that a brief interruption in the usual responsive care would be enough to cause insecure attachment and permanently raised stress levels.

However, I have also had numerous parents contact me having tried it and tell me that as well as it being extremely difficult to hear their baby crying, after more than a week of being consistent, there was no improvement in sleep. Furthermore, several parents have told me that they noticed changes in their baby's behaviour – such as their child being more irritable or clingy, or that their baby had stopped smiling in the day. I have also had numerous parents of toddlers contact me. They are often advised to leave their child to cry-it-out, and do so. For whatever reason, the improvement in sleep is not always permanent for these children, so they then have a choice – repeat the cry-it-out, or try something else. I've had parents tell me that they tried to repeat the intervention, only to find that their child was vomiting, or throwing themselves out of their cot, banging their head, or having anxiety before bedtime.

I'm not sure what makes the process 'easier' for some babies and children, and long, drawn-out and extreme for others. I suspect it is related to multiple factors – including internal resilience, parental stress, prenatal exposure to stress, individual stress response, attachment, temperament, personality and many other variables. The tricky thing is, that it is probably impossible to *predict* how children will respond. There are probably too many factors to assess, including some which *cannot* be assessed, for this to be an option. This is why I do not use it as a strategy at all. If I cannot prove it is definitely going to be safe for all children, then I won't take the risk.

Crying and resilience

When it comes to crying, we need to keep a sensible perspective. Babies cry for many reasons. Some of these we need to be concerned about and others we may need to accept as part of the fabric and soundtrack of raising children. It is unrealistic to think that if we are always emotionally available and responsive, babies will never cry. Certainly, we can reduce or eliminate crying that is brought about purely by being left alone. But what about the babies who cry in their car seat while you're driving down the motorway and cannot do anything about it? The babies who cry during illness? The babies who cry when they need to be left for 90 seconds because their parent simply *has* to use the bathroom? Babies who cry for hours during colicky phases? These babies are not going to be emotionally scarred by these experiences. In fact, children build resilience by being exposed to small amounts of stress that is then resolved.

I once saw a man and a little boy walking down the steps to the Underground in London. I didn't know them and doubt I'll ever see them again, but unwittingly they provided me with a beautiful metaphor I will never forget. The boy was carrying a heavy-looking backpack. The adult with him – who may or may not have been his father – could obviously see that the backpack was in danger of making the boy lose his balance as he came down the long flight of steps. But rather than take the boy's backpack from him, he simply lifted it at the top to reduce the weight to almost nothing. Once they were at the bottom of the steps, he gently released the backpack, allowing the boy to take its weight again. This is *exactly* what we need to do to build resilience. We do not *take* burdens from our children, we *help* them with their burdens until they are in a position to carry them alone.

Stress is thought to become toxic when it is prolonged, repeated or extreme.[32] Essentially, finding something stressful is not necessarily problematic in and of itself, but consistently being put in a stressful situation without parental support could be. Of course there are other factors – such as the emotional availability of another caring adult, the presence of a secure attachment, a child's prenatal exposures, and other buffers. Even in the womb, babies are exposed to stress, but when the stress is resolved, the infant's stress levels reduce as well. This is in fact their first lesson in resilience – that stress is not permanent.

Keeping a sensible perspective

Babies don't have too many options when it comes to communicating their needs. They need to be able to get our attention quickly and effectively. Before they have the command of language they can either use gestures or vocalisations. How sophisticated that vocalisation becomes is a developmental variable. As babies develop, they gradually begin making other noises rather than crying in order to get the response they need. We obviously need to be concerned about babies who are left to cry or crying when the cause cannot be determined. But is all crying bad? Certainly not.

Not responding to every little noise is one of those grey areas, and is highly subjective. It can feel controversial because it can be interpreted differently by different people. One person may describe a sound as a grizzle, another may perceive it as fussing, and someone else may interpret it as crying. Some studies find that infants sleep better when their genuine distress is responded to promptly, yet non-distress noises (whatever those are) are not responded to.[33] This is one of those suggestions that can be hard to get right – after all, interpreting different infant noises is not easy. I believe parents are the best judges of this. We have all heard our babies making squeaking, grumbling or grunting noises. These are easier to differentiate between than different 'types' of crying, which can be harder to discern in the early days.

We need to remember that there are different types of crying, and different types of stress as well. What we want to avoid is toxic stress.[34] Brief exposure to stress, with the emotional availability of an adult to provide support scaffolding to a child, is actually really beneficial and promotes resilience.[35] It is okay to have different types of response depending on the level of distress – in fact, that is what responsive parenting is all about: moderating our response in proportion to our children's needs.

In the safety of their parent's calm presence, children are able to learn that stress is not permanent, and that there are ways of managing, coping with and resolving stress. We do not need to be fearful about *all* crying causing stress that is harmful. As with so many other aspects of parenting, the balance can be hard to figure out. For now, I suggest that you try strategies that you feel comfortable with and that involve your presence.

The tired parent's summary

- Crying it out, and modified versions of it, are still popular strategies, and often discussed among child and healthcare professionals, parents and sleep researchers.
- The central debate is whether leaving children to cry alone may cause harm, either immediately or in the future. Many studies have been done to try to answer this question, and none of them are perfect – so we still have lots of unanswered questions.
- There are many grey areas within crying, and not all crying is bad. Crying can elicit a stress response from parents, and different cries are often interpreted as different needs. There is no simple answer that can be generalised to every baby.
- Many of the studies in recent years have measured circadian cortisol, instead of the stress response cortisol level. While these are related, they are separate mechanisms and we do not yet know how tightly these are related.
- Early, responsive, sensitive parenting promotes optimal development of the stress response system.
- Securely attached children generally sleep better, though secure attachment is not a panacea against fragmented sleep.
- It is difficult to predict which children may be more vulnerable to being left to cry – this may relate to their individual temperament, resilience and other protective factors such as genetics, the level of their stress response and their significant relationships with others.

Chapter ten

How to gently optimise your child's sleep

$\rightarrow$ 'Now you're talking', I hear you say. For anyone who has flipped straight to this chapter – I can completely understand that. You're tired. You want to know how to help your little one sleep as well as they possibly can. I totally get it. I'm going to be honest with you straight away though: *there is no super-easy, quick, cry-free way of getting your baby to stay asleep*. You're probably well aware of that, but I need to say it anyway. All I can do is throw a lot of gentle, evidence-based strategies at you and give you permission to decide which ones apply to your situation. None of these strategies involves leaving your baby to cry, leaving them alone, or denying them feeds – you don't need to do that in order to get better sleep.[1] Most of them involve a bit of groundwork, and you'll also need to discuss this with anyone else involved in caring for your baby. It's worth reading the sections for babies both older and younger than yours, as you'll probably be able to utilise some of those techniques as well.

Numerous studies suggest strategies that are reported to worsen sleep, as well as improve it. They are hard to compare and make sense of, since they all use different measurements, different definitions, different ages of children and rely on parental report.[2] The following suggestions are a round-up of completely safe ideas.

How to support your baby in the first few weeks

Feeding

The first thing to prioritise in the early weeks is feeding. You'll spend most of your time feeding your baby, whether by breast or bottle, and getting this nailed early on will save you a lot of time and stress later. The tricky thing is that if the feeding isn't going well, because it's such a major part of your day, it can affect the whole day – sleep included. For example:

Leo is feeding round the clock. His breastfeeds are at least 50 minutes every time, and he wants to feed again less than an hour afterwards. He's fussy and doesn't sleep more than about five minutes on his own, so his parents are holding him most of the time, day and night.

Nia is bottle-fed, and is fussy at every feed. She takes a long time to feed – at least 45 minutes, is very windy and cries a lot in between. She also spits up. She will only sleep bolt upright.

Both of these babies have feeding problems that are impacting their behaviour and sleep. It is inappropriate to consider these as sleep problems – the root cause is feeding-related. Getting to the bottom of the frequent, fussy and inefficient feeding will almost certainly improve the overall feel and flow of their day.

Feeding is sometimes completely smooth sailing from the first day, but for most people, it's something they need to work on and get support with. Responsively feeding your baby, whether you are breast or bottle-feeding, will mean your baby learns to manage their appetite, doesn't get stressed during or in between feeds, and will get the right amount of milk.

Ways to help

Breastfed babies	Bottle-fed babies	All babies
Get help with the positioning (latch)	Practise paced bottle-feeding	Feed your baby when they show early feeding cues
Find someone who can teach you how to be sure your baby is feeding effectively	Don't let too many people get involved with feeding – it's a lovely bonding experience for parents	Offer babies a chance to burp and have some upright time after feeds

The early days and weeks are a time to enjoy and get to know your baby. There is no evidence that feeding babies on a schedule will help them sleep, and these schedules may be hard to follow for most babies. A recent study found that they only worked for about 15 percent of babies, and when they didn't work, parents were more likely to become depressed.[3] Feeding your baby when they ask to be fed, allowing them to feed for as long as they want, and stopping when they want, is likely to be less stressful for you and your baby. The only exception to this is if your baby is not waking up frequently, when you may need to wake them. Ask your health professional if you're not sure.

Closeness, responsiveness and attachment

Feeding and responsiveness often go hand in hand. There is actually good evidence that promoting strong parent-child attachment optimises sleep.[4-6] You really can't cuddle or hold your baby too much. I have found time and time again that when parents and babies just enjoy spending time together in an unhurried fashion, without feeling like they are getting it wrong, or 'making a rod for their back', they feel less stressed. The less stressed you are, the more you'll enjoy parenting. That doesn't mean you'll love every minute. It doesn't mean you won't have times when you miss your child-free days. But just slowing down and accepting that these days are likely to be full of sitting around and not getting much done besides looking after yourself and your baby will take the pressure off.

Responsiveness means that you match your response to the level of need your little one has.[7] That means that if your baby is perfectly content lying in their crib, or on the floor looking at shadows, it's totally fine to do something else for a short while. You don't need to have your baby constantly in your arms in order to define responsiveness. Don't feel guilty! If your baby is chewing a toy and seems perfectly happy, and you need to get dinner started, then that's fine. If, however, your baby is having a day when they're only happy in your arms, then use a baby carrier and keep them with you as you get on with your day. We don't want to ignore babies when they have needs, but we don't have to over-parent when they are content.

I wish I could give you a magic key to having a baby who is content and calm most of the time. I can't though. Some babies are naturally relaxed and easy-going from the beginning. Others seem to be on high alert and don't switch off. This means that some babies will need you more than others. This is not your fault – don't let anyone tell you that your baby needs you more because you've been more available to them. It's simply not true. Babies learn to be more independent by first having their needs for dependence met – in other words, if you consistently prioritise close, caring, comfort for your baby, you will build a strong attachment. When children are securely attached, they feel more confident to leave you – because they know you will always be there if they need you. Anyone who says anything different is not up to date.

This type of care is not just great for bonding and attachment. There is actually plenty of research that demonstrates that responsive feeding and parenting, high warmth and emotional availability throughout the day and at bedtime aids sleep, and is associated with better sleep consolidation.[8-10]

What you can do
There are so many ways to develop a close bond with your child:

- Cuddles and holding
- Babywearing
- Co-bathing
- Massage
- Reading stories, singing songs, telling nursery rhymes
- Dancing with them
- Going for a walk and telling them about the things you see
- Talking to them while you go about your day
- Letting them be a part of whatever you're doing

Babies don't need vast numbers of toys. They often have no interest in soft toys and stuffed animals in the early weeks. They don't want fancy play gyms or to watch baby DVDs. You are literally their favourite person, and they would happily spend all day with you, just watching whatever you're doing.

How others can help

If you're a family member or friend – thank you for taking the time to read this. There is so much you can do to help. Here are a few ideas:

- Ask when the best time to visit is, and bring food
- Set up a 'meal train' so that other people in the family's friendship circle and community can coordinate bringing meals for the new family
- Stock up the fridge and freezer with easy-to-grab nutritious food that needs very little preparation
- Organise a cleaning roster
- Instead of (or as well as!) buying presents and toys, have everyone chip in and hire a postnatal doula
- Offer to care for other children, walk the dog or clean out the rabbit hutch
- Sit and listen, offer words of encouragement and reassurance
- Offer to sit and cuddle the baby for an hour while the new parents go out for a quick bite to eat, or a coffee

Getting support is so important in the early days. You have a lot to adjust to – becoming a parent and adapting to the new dynamic in your relationship with your partner can be a lot to take in, alongside trying to feed, care for and bond with your baby. Make it a personal goal to not turn down any offers of help. People aren't judging how self-sufficient you are. They *want* to help. Trust me. If you don't let them – you're actually denying them the joy of being able to give back, and get closer to you. Being vulnerable is hard, but I guarantee that if you can let your walls down and allow others to be there for you, you'll find this easier, and you may have closer friends as well.

Circadian rhythm

If you've stuck with me faithfully so far, this will probably come as no surprise. You can really give your little one a head start by exposing them to as much natural daylight as possible,[11] especially first thing in the morning.[12] If your baby or child is older and you're reading this section to glean little nuggets of wisdom, then it's never too late to start to do this. The weather doesn't have to be perfect either – all outdoor light counts, not just beautiful balmy sunny skies. Get outdoors as much as possible – light is the principal environmental cue that will set your baby's body clock.

The other cues are noise, social cues and activity levels. For older children, eating at regular and consistent times is also important. Try to make no adaptations to your noise or activity levels in the day – this helps your baby learn the difference between night and day. This can be hard if it's your first baby – many of us simply don't make that much noise! If this is you, try playing music in the day, or keep the radio on as background noise. Don't tiptoe around! Sometimes people do this instinctively. I remember one day my daughter's classmate brought his ducklings into school for the class to enjoy (cutest thing you've ever seen, for the record). The children all spoke in hushed voices around the ducklings. Their class teacher – himself a fairly recent new parent – made no effort to correct them. After all, the peace and quiet was a welcome change from the usual chaos of six-year-olds *en masse*! However, for human babies, there is no need to keep things hushed.

Multiple sleep cues

One final tip is for *how* you get your baby to fall asleep. There is nothing wrong with however you help your baby settle and sleep. In these early weeks, your baby will fall asleep quite automatically – you do not 'teach' them to fall asleep. They simply will. They may fall asleep in your arms, while you feed them, in the pram/stroller, the car – you name it. There's not only nothing wrong with that, but there's also not much you can do about it either! Do not waste a single moment of emotional energy worrying about this. However, if you felt you wanted to be proactive, one simple and gentle strategy you could use is to overlay multiple sleep cues, rather than become dependent on one single cue. This goes back to the idea of habit stacking. For example, if you find your baby tends to fall asleep feeding most of the time, then consider patting or stroking your baby or gently humming or singing at the same time. Think of it as your sleep switch. If the switch you always press to get your baby to sleep is feeding, then while this isn't a problem *per se*, it means that if at some point you decide you'd rather not rely solely on one sleep switch, you have several that your little one associates with sleep. I often recommend offering multiple sleep cues that touch on several different senses. A sleep cue you can feel (stroking, touching, patting), a sleep cue you can hear (shushing, singing, humming, deep breathing), and a sleep cue you can smell (diffuser in the room, a sheet or muslin square that smells like a parent). You could also consider rocking or feeding as other cues as well. Further down the line, this means that if you decide to stop rocking or feeding, for example, you have only taken away one cue out of the four that your baby is familiar with. It makes everyone's life easier.

After the first few weeks

Teamwork, co-parenting and social support

After the first few adrenaline-fuelled weeks, fatigue can begin to set in, just as the visitors start to become less frequent. You'll need to plan your social support so that you still have company, friendship, practical help and emotional scaffolding. There is good evidence that promoting and encouraging teamwork among parents is independently associated with better sleep.[13,14] Have open and honest conversations with your partner about how you're each coping. Perhaps arrange to 'check in' with someone who will listen – whether that is your partner, a friend or a family member. Having a safe space where you can emotionally offload is really important. Remember that co-parenting works best when there is a shared experience of the highs and lows, free from criticism or dismissal of concerns by the other parent. If you have a supportive partnership already, make it a priority to invest in your partner to prevent it from being neglected with the demands of parenting. If your partnership could use some work, then don't delay – get some help with this, and you're likely to reap the benefits with a more rewarding relationship, better mental health and improvements in sleep for everyone.

It has also been found that children who grow up in a supportive family environment sleep better and have more consolidated sleep.[15] Make family time your priority from the beginning. Even before your baby can eat solid food, make it a habit to sit down together, debrief the day, share the successes and challenges and make time for each other. There is no better time to start a habit than as soon as possible.

Finally, support scaffolding is sometimes necessary for families who are struggling. I encourage you to reach out to your social, community, and family networks wherever possible. If it is a financially viable option for you, then paid support can help you to feel more on top of things.[16] This may look different for every family – consider what you're finding difficult. Different tasks that could potentially be outsourced include:

- Shopping – could your partner do this on their way home? Or online shopping?
- Postnatal doulas can be hugely helpful to offer support, guidance and reassurance without 'taking over'
- Someone to come over in the evening if you struggle with this time of the day to offer either practical help – such as another pair of hands for bath time – or emotional support when you're feeling tired and emotional. This could be a neighbour, friend, or even a local teen who wants to earn some extra cash
- A cleaner, or someone to deal with the laundry
- A dog-walker
- Someone to mow the grass and tidy up the garden

Sometimes people will offer to do tasks that you actually enjoy – keep those to yourself. Outsource tasks that drive you crazy instead. If you hate laundry and have the means to pass it on to a launderette – do it. If you love your dog but feel guilty that you can't walk her, find a neighbour or go to a website that matches people who want to borrow dogs with people who need occasional doggy daycare. There is almost always something that you can boot off your to-do list without the need to let everything go to ruin. Just reducing the number of jobs can make your remaining jobs feel less overwhelming.

Consistency and bedtime routines

This isn't going to win any prizes for originality, but it is well known that consistency in general, as well as providing a consistent bedtime routine, is associated with more sleep.[17] I tend to think about this in multiple ways – consistency might mean different things in different contexts. For example, consistency of responsiveness does not mean that you always provide the same response. If your child is mildly upset your response will be different than if they are very distressed. What is consistent is that you provide the right level of response each time. However, at other times, doing more or less the same thing is really helpful. This is also true of a bedtime routine. Having a consistent, positive bedtime routine is known to have a dose-response effect – that is, the more you use your bedtime routine and the more consistent it is, the more it seems to be associated with a stress-free bedtime.[18] Bedtime routines are sometimes misunderstood.

How to help

Things to try	Things to avoid
• Anything soothing • 3–4 activities that you and your baby enjoy • Doing the same activities in the same order • Be willing to be flexible about the exact timings – some days your child may be more or less tired • Try a mini version of your bedtime routine for naps	• Anything that upsets your child – stress is counter-productive for sleep • A very long bedtime routine tends to lose focus, and your baby may get a second wind • A very short bedtime routine may not be long enough for your baby to calm down • Strict timings

You can and should observe your baby and do what works for you both. If a bath gets your little one stressed out and fretful – scrap it, or try it earlier in the day. If books get thrown across the room, or chewed, then leave them and try something else. Just because 'bath, massage, PJs, two stories, lights out' works for your friend, or worked for your eldest child, doesn't mean it will work for your little one. Don't be afraid to experiment, and when you find what works, stick with it.

One tricky area to get right is the length of the routine. I'm not going to suggest how long this should be because I don't know your baby's age, temperament, attention span or family dynamic. All I will say is that the bedtime routine is like an express train to 'sleepytown'. You don't want the train to get derailed or diverted too much. Keep it simple and succinct, with not too many stops on the way.

Stress management and emotional wellbeing

I spend a lot of time talking about 'emotion contagion'. This is a fascinating phenomenon whereby you can influence others with your own emotional state.[19] It is not just about copying facial expressions and mirroring responses, though this is also important,[20,21] but actually causing another person to unconsciously mimic your emotional state. This is great news, because as long as you're aware of this, you can use it to your advantage. If you can project calm, positivity and confidence about sleep, your little one is more likely to be calm and confident as well. Now, you may be thinking that sleep is a flashpoint – a bone of contention that makes you frustrated or angry. That's a good place to start. Recognise how sleep makes you feel, and then you may be able to deal with those feelings. You're not a bad person for finding sleep annoying. In fact, you'd have to be a saint not to be frustrated at least some of the time about children's sleep habits. But the trick is to do something constructive about how you feel. Emotionally 'park' the feelings somewhere. Write them down. Say them out loud, or call a friend. Keep a diary, or punch a pillow. Repeat affirmations or practise guided relaxation or mindfulness. Use an app, YouTube or simply read out your affirmation until you feel calmer. Another trick is to try alternate nostril yoga breathing. This is an amazingly calming and quick self-help tool that has been shown to lower your heart rate and respiratory rate.[22] Here's how you do it:

1. Half pinch your nose so that your right nostril is blocked
2. Exhale through the unblocked left nostril and then inhale through the left
3. Block the left and exhale through the right
4. Inhale through the right, then block the left

It sounds more complicated than it really is. Give it a try – it's completely harmless, subtle, and can be done anywhere, with no equipment. Just bringing your awareness to your breath, and consciously slowing down your breathing, while thinking positively may be enough to make you feel calmer, and thus calm your baby. Try the following affirmations:

- How well my baby sleeps will not define me as a parent
- It is not my responsibility to make my child fall asleep, all I can do is provide the opportunity
- Sleep will come one day
- Sleep may be hard today, but there are things I can work on
- I am a calm, confident, compassionate parent
- My baby is lucky to have me, and I am lucky to have them

Just by taking 5–10 minutes to get control of your emotions and breathing may make a huge difference, not only to your baby, but also to your confidence level.

Feeling confident in your ability to parent seems to be positively linked to a better judgement of the level of response needed by infants, and consequent better sleep.[23] It appears that worrying about sleep is often linked with poorer sleep, while less anxiety about sleep, realistic expectations about sleep, and feeling good about your parenting leads to better infant sleep. I suspect this self-fulfilling prophecy is a combination of both emotions and behaviours. If you are feeling worried, stressed or anxious, you may be more likely to be very vigilant, and over-parent. On the other hand, if you can recognise this and get some help for it, you are likely to be more relaxed, feel confident in both yourself and your baby, and more appropriately responsive.

Understanding your baby's cues

Another area to work on is being observant of your baby's cues and responding to their individual tiredness levels.[24] I'm sometimes asked for examples of what babies might do when they are tired. This is very variable, and while yawning, fussing, losing interest in toys or crying are cues for some babies, for others there may be completely different ones. I seem to spend a lot of time instead helping parents think about observing their baby's emotional state, curiosity, and willingness to explore and engage throughout the day, and in different environments and contexts. A really transformative piece of work is the *Zones of Regulation*.[25] This is a way of recognising and responding to your child's energy and emotional state to avoid them becoming dysregulated. 'Scaling' the level of distress in this way helps parents to moderate their response to meet the child's needs.

- Blue: your little one may be tired, lethargic or sleepy
- Green: this means good to go! Calm, peaceful and energised children reside in the green zone
- Yellow: worried, anxious, mildly stressed or nervous little people
- Red: this is how we feel when we are angry, extremely over-excited, or distressed. Meltdowns and uncontrollable behaviour happen from the red zone

You will need to pay attention and notice what triggers your child to go from green to yellow, or yellow back to green. How do you get them from yellow to blue? And what strategies do you only haul out when they are red?

For example, rocking may only be needed during certain times. During a meltdown or inconsolable crying, deep pressure – such as firm massage, tight hugs, swaddling or wrapping in a sheet may be more helpful than rocking or bouncing or shushing. You might not need to do this more than once in a while. By paying attention to what works and when, and what the triggers are, you can work out what your baby needs and at what time. The goals are to spot patterns of behaviour, so you can learn to be more attuned to the needs of your child in particular states. It's tempting to think of the red zone as a no-go area. In truth, that is unrealistic. We all see red from time to time. Negative emotions are normal – the goal is to learn how to handle them positively. For sleep, you'll need to learn how your child gets into the blue zone.

Paying attention to your child's emotional state will also help you to avoid excessive sleep pressure.[26] This is important so that your baby naps at a time that is good for them in terms of their energy level and emotional regulation. When a baby misses their window to go to sleep they can become fretful and more unsettled. It's important to remember, however, that the world will not come crashing down if your baby has a bad nap day. Honestly, if your baby misses a nap now and then, you will all manage. Don't let it rule or ruin your day.

Sensory input

There is some suggestion that infants who have 'higher need' temperaments and also poor sleep may have a single underlying sensory need. This is not to suggest that they have a disorder, but simply have sensory needs that are not met. Everyone has a different sensory profile. Do you have a sensitive sense of smell? Or do you feel pain less acutely than your partner? Do you become irritated by a sticky sensation on your hands? Or are you oblivious to it? Many people are becoming more aware of diagnoses like sensory processing disorder, so I am always mindful that when I talk about sensory needs, I do not want people to become anxious that I mean a sensory disorder. For a small proportion of people, this is the case, but everyone has sensory preferences – there's nothing remotely pathological about that. Working out what your baby prefers may help you to meet their needs better, and lead to better attunement between you and them, as well as more settled behaviour and better sleep.

For example, if an infant is hypersensitive to noise and lives in a noisy environment, then this would not only make them irritable, but also likely to startle to loud or breakthrough noises. If an infant is sensitive to textures, then a scratchy label in their clothing, or wearing fabric that makes them sweat may make them fussy and also resist sleep due to discomfort. Thus, getting to the bottom of whatever is the underlying cause of the fussy behaviour may also improve sleep.[27-29] This is all part of the need to assess babies and children individually. The best person to do that is you.

Some generalisations to start you off while you work out the specifics for your little one:

- Most babies are more comfortable in 100 percent cotton clothing
- It's never going to be a bad idea to avoid labels, applique patches, or buttons/poppers down the back of an outfit
- If your baby hates baths, consider what it is that they hate – is it water in their eyes? The temperature? Are they too tired when they go in the bath? Are the lights too bright?
- Most babies enjoy deep pressure. Only some babies enjoy light, feathery, tickly touch

It's a mistake to assume that all babies like the same things. Sometimes we are recommended to try certain activities, only to find that this is precisely what is exacerbating the problem. For example:

Josh's unsettled behavior was really getting to Ada. Ada was beginning to complain of backache from bouncing Josh to sleep for every nap. Ada found that Josh would only sleep if she firmly bounced him up and down, while standing up. Josh would cry and squirm throughout and would eventually fall asleep in her arms.

The problem had started when Josh was a very young baby and did not seem to sleep as much as his peers. Ada became concerned that he wasn't getting enough sleep. She had assumed that Josh was tired but resisting sleep, and spoke to a friend who suggested bouncing him. Ada tried this and it worked first time. She then (quite understandably) thought that Josh needed to be bounced in order to fall asleep, so assumed the responsibility for getting him to sleep.

What probably happened was that she got lucky the first time, or Josh happened to be tired when she tried. But as time went on, Josh didn't need to sleep every time Ada was trying to get him to sleep, and rather than trust her instinct and her baby, she was made anxious by comparing him to other babies. Bouncing to sleep was not what Josh needed, which was why it was so difficult to get him to fall asleep this way, and why he cried and squirmed.

When I met Ada, she felt hopeless, worried and angry. She was frustrated that her baby was so 'resistant' to falling asleep, even though he 'really needed to sleep', and was becoming resentful about how much effort it took to get him to sleep, and how painful her back and hips were getting now that he was older and heavier. She was also becoming doubtful of her own parenting competence and instinct. In this situation, Ada needed a massive dose of self-confidence and to begin to learn how to read Josh's cues in the day. Ada loved the zones of regulation, as they helped her to be able to give Josh what he needed, rather than what her friends or strict sleep books said he needed. Once she was able to watch Josh and follow his lead when he seemed to be in the blue zone, she found that he didn't need bouncing at all. She simply lay down beside him and he went to sleep. No stress. No backache.

The moral of the story is that your baby is a genius. They will tell you what they need if you can trust your baby and your instincts. I'm not saying that instinct is always innate – in fact, I've known many people who feel they need to really work at learning what their baby's cues mean, but if you can develop the ability to be open-minded, and not be led by other people's experiences or expectations, it will really help you.

After six months

The first thing to say at the six-month point is – you're doing really well, keep going! If you were holding on to the hope that at six months your baby would sleep through, and they aren't, then take heart: you're in good company. I mention this fact a lot, but more than 70 percent of babies aged 6-18 months wake up more than once a night. If your baby sleeps through, you are in the very fortunate minority.

Practical considerations

Some of the difficulties of this age are logistical. Fitting in naps, solid food, playtime and household tasks can be really challenging. They don't say parenting is a full-time job for nothing. If you're feeling the strain at this point – you're not alone. A lot of parents reflect that when their babies were very young, they assumed that everything would get easier. It's a natural tendency to look forward to the next big thing – whether that is sitting up, crawling, or eating solid food. We sometimes assume that these major milestones will be the key to better sleep. 'When this tooth comes through, it will get better', 'When she's finally able to sit she'll be happier to sit on the floor and play', 'When he can crawl he won't be so frustrated', 'When we start solids, it might help'. The truth is that kids are constantly changing. I don't mean to burst anyone's bubble, but usually one milestone passing is the cue for another phase to start.

I wish someone had told me early on that parenting doesn't necessarily get any easier, it just changes. That is not supposed to sound negative. Parenting is wonderful, hilarious, challenging and rewarding – not all the time of course, but it *is* all those things, at least sometimes. It is also extremely hard work, and sometimes requires the tact and diplomacy of the peace corps, the logistical precision of a military expedition, and the patience of a saint. If you are finding it difficult – know that it will change. Soon. Your situation may be replaced by a different and equally challenging issue, but it will not stay the same, that's for sure.

Some practical tips that have been shared with me over the years include:

- Always have snacks and a drink in every bag you have (for you and your baby!).
- Bring a change of clothes everywhere. There's nothing more frustrating than having to leave a fun activity because your little one has smeared broccoli and tomato pasta literally all over themselves, or a nappy explosion has made them a social outcast.
- Work out what your immovable daily anchors are. Everything else can be flexible around them. For example, you could make mealtimes consistent (to within a reasonable degree of flexibility of course), but activities, outings, playtime and chores can be slotted in wherever they fit.
- Plan to spend no more than half the day at home – you and your baby are very likely to get bored.
- Try to have the easiest nap at home – use this one to catch up on what you want to do.

- Maintain a loose structure at the beginning and end of the day. I often suggest allowing for a 'grace period' so that bedtime can be earlier or later by about 30 minutes if your little one is very tired, or conversely, if you are busy, or they are not tired.

Naps

After six months, most babies settle into a slightly more predictable pattern of napping, thanks to the full maturation of their circadian rhythm. Depending on their age, they will most likely have 2–3 naps, but as always, your baby may buck the trend and do their own thing. If it works for you and them – leave it alone. One tip that is very consistently found in most studies is to refrain from later afternoon naps after about 7–8 months, as these can have a negative effect on nighttime sleep – as can too much daytime sleep in general.[30]

If your evenings and nights have gone belly up it is worth reviewing your naps and daytimes in general. Is your little one having enough daytime sleep? Is it too much? There's nothing wrong with experimenting to see if longer awake windows between sleep opportunities improve the situation, or reducing the number of naps, trying alternate locations for naps, or bringing bedtime earlier or later. If you do decide to make a change, try to only change one thing at a time, so you can make a sensible decision about what has made an impact and what hasn't. Another good rule of thumb is to try anything for several days before deciding to abandon it as a lost cause. Don't forget – habits are not born overnight. If one day of two naps instead of three makes absolutely no difference, don't write it off immediately. Persevere for a few days before deciding one way or the other. I meet many people who try multiple different strategies every couple of days, only to find that they have become frustrated and confused about what works and what doesn't.

Co-parenting

Involvement of fathers with their children, specifically providing more frequent emotional support, is associated with better sleep, and this is a long-term finding. In one study, fathers who were more involved at age two had children who slept better at age three, suggesting that this is related to the long-term father-child relationship.[31] Other research suggests that same-sex parents are more likely to have a more equal division of care and household chores, which leads to less conflict. The bottom line is that caring for children and homes is hard work, and can cause tension. Find a way of sharing the load and you're likely to reduce the stress. Finding ways of facilitating close relationships with and between both parents, if there are two, is also really important for children's emotional well-being and sleep.[32]

Activities, stimulation and calm-down time

During the day, your baby or child needs to have an ebb and flow. Giving the day more oscillating energy can help a child switch from one state to the next. If they go from quiet play to a quiet walk, to calmly interacting with parents, to a calm-down time before bed, you might find that they resist falling asleep. It's not that you've done anything wrong, they perhaps have just been a bit stuck in the blue zone.

I spend a lot of time discussing stress management and the need to remain calm – it's hard to go from a high-energy tickle fight or chasing game straight into bedtime.[33] But adding in energy and dynamics to your baby's day is also crucial for sleep. The ideal situation is some movement between the green zone and yellow zone for some excitement, into a calm-down time which eases a child into sleep. I often meet parents who are instigating a really lovely calming bedtime routine. They might have a bath in a dimly-lit room, a massage, story, cuddle and into bed. And then sleep doesn't follow. What's that about? Well, we don't want to do such a good job of keeping things calm, that we end up with a day that lacks fun and pace.

It is hard for a baby or child to calm down for bedtime, when they've essentially been *calm all day*. It's boring! It's like your baby is on cruise control, drifting in the same energy state for different activities. You can end up with a day that lacks stimulation. In fact, the appropriate amount of stimulation at home seems to contribute to optimal sleep-wake states of prematurely born babies.[34]

I'm not talking about scheduling fun here, but planning in fun activities, alongside time for your child to just co-exist with you and whatever you're doing, and some one-to-one interaction time is really important. I often suggest what I call 'silly time' before bedtime. This might sound like madness, but children build up stresses and frustrations throughout the day. Big belly laughing, lots of movement and activity will give them a chance to get their pent-up frustrations and excess energy out of their system. This is a great time to involve a partner who has just got in from work. Many families find this works really well, provided it suits their child. Then allow for 20 minutes to calm down before you start preparing your child for going to sleep.

Sleep hygiene

If you've not already given this an overhaul, now is a good time. With solid food a factor, as well as activities and differentiation between night and day, this is a good age to make sure you've tried all the obvious tricks to help your little one's circadian rhythm. A healthy lifestyle, including diet, exercise, emotional wellbeing and stress management have all been shown to optimise sleep naturally.[35,36] Diet could be a whole book in itself, but the bottom line is to try to remember that it is your job to offer a range of healthy, nutritious food that your baby is developmentally capable of handling, and it is your baby's job to decide whether and how much of it they will eat. Try to offer foods from every colour of the rainbow, and remember that your baby's tummy is only about the size of their fist – they may want to eat little and often.

Some people look at me strangely when I talk about exercise in a pre-walking baby. I'm not suggesting that your little nine-month old does 10 push-ups every day, but there are lots of ways to wear your little people out physically. Only 50-100 years ago, everyone got a lot more exercise purely because they would have walked to the shops, school and work. Cars were a luxury and expensive to run (frankly they still are, but we have absorbed this into our normal way of life). We now need to consciously think of ways to be active, rather than this being an inherent part of our lives. Here are some fun ideas:

- Create a baby floor cushion obstacle course. Place rolled up blankets and pillows on the floor and encourage your little one to scramble and haul them themselves over and around the obstacles
- Have tickle fights on the floor
- Support your baby to walk by letting them hold on to your hands
- Encourage your baby to spend time on their tummy, pushing, wriggling, crawling or rolling around
- Try swimming – often this triggers a great nap
- With older babies and toddlers, allow them to walk as much as they can – plan for extra time so that you can let them walk
- Try a balance bike or mini scooter
- Dance around the house

Finally, there is a substantial amount of evidence to suggest that you avoid use of screens, artificial light, electronic devices, apps and gaming, particularly in the two hours before bedtime.[37] Lots of people wouldn't dream of exposing their babies to these gadgets directly, but some very sensitive babies are affected just by the TV being on ambiently in the room. Consider turning all devices off 1–2 hours before bedtime, as it can take about two hours for melatonin levels to begin to rise after the onset of dimmer lights.[38] Some research suggests that you reduce artificial light exposure even if it doesn't have an obvious immediate effect on children's sleep – it may increase REM sleep, which is not as restorative, and may lead to more awakenings with nightmares.[39]

At all ages, if you can work on the basics – attachment and connection, feeding, sleep hygiene, stress management, naps and sensory stimulation, sleep is more likely to come easily for you. By investing in your and your child's emotional wellbeing, getting support when you need it, and prioritising a responsive style of parenting, you'll know that you have set yourself up for the best possible sleep situation.

The tired parent's summary

- There are many theories about how to improve sleep and what may worsen sleep. Unfortunately, everyone uses different strategies, ages of children and research methods. This makes conclusions about what works best hard to draw.
- In the early weeks, prioritise feeding. Get lots of support until you feel you have this completely sorted, whether you are breast or bottle feeding, or both.
- It is definitely important to practise a responsive, loving style of parenting – this seems to optimise sleep in the long term.
- Get lots of support from your partner, friends and family in the early days. There are many ways for people to be involved and ease the fatigue of caring for a new baby.
- Expose young babies to plenty of natural daylight and do not minimise household noise.
- Try providing multiple cues for sleep so that from a young age, babies learn many ways to settle.
- Work as a team, support your co-parent and have open conversations about what support you need specifically.
- Develop a flexibly timed but positive and consistent bedtime routine.
- Look after your emotional wellbeing, minimise or manage your stress as best you can, and prioritise self-care.

- Learn to read your individual baby's cues for tiredness, boredom, hunger and other needs, rather than rely on prescribed sleep schedules.
- Pay attention to your child's emotional state and 'zones of regulation' to avoid them building up stress and tension during the day which may affect your night.
- For older babies, the logistics of fitting in play, solid food, naps and milk feeds can require some creativity and flexibility. Work around your immovable daily anchors, and provide a balance of activity and quiet time.
- During times of change, when sleep often becomes 'collateral damage', go back to basics and review naps, individual cues and manage your own emotional response.
- Work on sleep hygiene – your sleep environment, reducing screen time, increasing exercise, and optimising diet and mental health to passively improve sleep with very little effort.

Chapter eleven

Managing a sleep crisis with kindness

→ Are you in a sleep crisis? Or are you wondering what that looks like? Are you trying to understand what your options are and whether you might be able to prevent your sleep situation from becoming unsustainable? I meet a lot of families who have various different struggles and difficulties. Nobody's sleep story is the same, and yet there are always similarities, so you are by no means alone.

Let's start by working out where you are right now. Broadly speaking, I meet four categories of people with sleep struggles:

1. People who need some gentle reassurance.
2. People who need additional support.
3. People who need some simple sleep strategies.
4. People who would define their situation as a crisis.

While you might immediately identify with one of these categories, I'll try to give you some examples. The point of this is so that you get the support that is appropriate for you right now.

183

1. Gentle reassurance required

If this is you, deep down you know that your baby is normal. You might doubt yourself, but you fundamentally do not think you have a sleep problem. Perhaps you have had one too many negative comments about sleep. Maybe you feel that your little one doesn't nap like other babies, or perhaps you feel like the only parent who is feeding or rocking their baby to sleep. You might feel like you are under pressure to do something about your sleep situation. Let me tell you: you do not have to do anything you don't want to. If your baby's sleep is not bothering you deep down, it's not a problem. Sleep is never an issue just because someone or some book says it is. You are not spoiling your baby. You are badly in need of cheerleaders to tell you that you are awesome. Your baby is not broken, and you are doing the best possible thing by responding to them and keeping them close and calm.[1] Keep doing what you're doing.

If this resonates with you, find a way of drumming it in. Perhaps you need to find your sleep tribe? Do you need to unfollow a few Instagram accounts? Stop telling certain people you're tired because the only response they ever give is one you don't feel comfortable with? You'll need to surround yourself with people who can remind you of the things you need to hear. Online support, when it is a group that resonates with your values, can be a valuable social network.[2]

2. Additional support

If you need additional support, you are a parent who still feels that your baby is sleeping completely normally. You know that you're doing a great job and your baby is getting the very best start with your gentle responsive care.

Yet you feel like you are struggling to cope. You may lack the resources to keep going and feel like you are waving for help. You do not necessarily feel like you or you baby need 'fixing', but equally you know that you cannot keep going without something having to give.

If this is you, I urge you to be honest with someone. Please have the courage to be vulnerable. Do you have a partner you can talk to? A friend? Neighbour? Family member? Can you team up with another parent and look after their little one for an hour or two and then have them return the favour? Is paid support or additional childcare an option? Is there anything you can outsource?

3. Simple sleep strategies

If this is you, you have reached a point in your journey where you recognise that your sleep situation is becoming unsustainable and you want to take some steps to prevent it from overwhelming you. You may feel like you're coping well enough to take some proactive steps yourself, or you might feel like you need to take those steps alongside some additional support.

I want to reassure you that if this is you, you do not have to do anything scary, stressful or inconsistent with your parenting style. There are so many things you can do to get yourself to a point where you feel you can cope well. What is it that you are specifically finding hard? Days or nights? Is it one nap in particular? Is it just bedtime? Is it night waking? Be as specific as you can, and work on the activities that are most likely to improve the area you are struggling with. If it's more than one, don't worry – just work on one area at a time if you like. There is no rule about needing to tackle everything at once.

4. Sleep crisis

If this is you, you'll know it before you've finished reading the paragraph. This is an unsustainable and unmanageable situation. Parents often use language that is quite desperate: 'I can't take it anymore', 'I'm going to die from lack of sleep', 'I've thought of walking out', 'I'll do anything'.

You feel like you stopped waving a long time ago. You now feel like you're drowning and are desperate for help. You may feel conflicted and guilty that you're struggling to cope. You may even wonder how you're going to get out of this situation because you're so tired that the thought of doing anything about your child's sleep is deeply intimidating.

I meet a lot of people who feel stuck when they get to this point. They know, deep down, that although they are desperate for things to change, the thought of making any change feels daunting. The reason for this is that whatever you're currently doing is likely to be the:

- Easiest
- Quickest, and
- Most reliable way of getting your little one back to sleep

Doing *anything* else then, by definition, is likely to be *harder, slower and less reliable*.

You may be in a crisis because of some contextual factor such as ill-health or mental health struggle. Maybe your strategy worked in the early days – but now not so much. You may have a family situation or a problem with another child that means you are struggling to cope. You may feel like you could deal with this if you had a live-in nanny, cleaner, cook and PA, but since you don't, it is categorically unmanageable.

If you are in a crisis, you still don't need to leave your baby to cry. Even an emergency doesn't mean that you need to lower your standards and accept options that you previously thought were unacceptable. You still need to prioritise gentleness and responsiveness and reassurance. You might need to make some changes. Don't worry, there are lots of ideas coming up.

Simple sleep strategies first

Whether you only need to do this, or you're in a crisis, this is the first step. In fact, many families are deeply encouraged by the fact that they don't need to do *all the things*, or tackle everything at once. Remember the step-by-step approach to sleep:

- You can get your child to sleep at a time that works for them, using any means necessary, in any place that will work
- You can get your child to sleep at a time that works for them, using any means necessary, with some limits on location that work for you
- You can get your child to sleep at a time that works for them, using any means necessary, in the location that works for you
- You can get your child to sleep at a time that works for them, with the support and location that works for you

This means that you need only focus on one specific area to improve. For example:

Autumn had reached breaking point with her 10-month-old son Hunter. She had recently split from her partner of 12 years, and had understandably been feeling stressed. She has Crohn's disease which tends to flare up with stress. Because of the split, she was financial-

ly under pressure to return to her job doing project work. Hunter was taking more than an hour to fall asleep at bedtime, after his bedtime routine, and then was awake every 40 minutes. He napped just twice a day, but never longer than 20 minutes. When Autumn called me, she was tearful and desperate, and was describing feeling completely trapped because she wanted to be able to get work done in the evening, so Hunter's sleep habits were a source of great anxiety. She described her goal of being able to put him down in his cot and have him fall asleep peacefully. Yet this felt overwhelming. Starting with observing his awake windows and sleep cues, Autumn was able to alter naps to suit Hunter better. She also made Hunter's bedtime a little later, when he showed signs of genuine tiredness, which had an instant effect on his sleep. Having a plan to work towards helped her anxiety, and bedtimes began to improve. If Autumn had tried to tackle everything, including nights, at this point, when she was physically and emotionally fragile, the chances are she would have found it too hard, which could potentially have added to her stress or worsened her self-esteem.

Given that you do not have to tackle everything, you may need to decide what to address first. You could consider any of the following areas to work on:

- Are there any underlying factors that could be causing the problem – such as a feeding issue, health problem, reflux or allergy? Do you need to book a doctor's appointment? Would it help to call an IBCLC or go along to a breastfeeding drop-in?
- Prioritise your emotional health and wellbeing. This includes stress management, mental health problems, trauma and anxiety. Do you need to see your doctor, counsellor or psychotherapist?
- What do you wish someone would say to you? Imagine the person you respect most in the world. If that person could say one thing that would boost your self-esteem and sense of parenting self-efficacy – what would it be? 'You're amazing', 'You're enough', 'You're an incredible parent', 'You're doing a great job'. This becomes your positive affirmation. Repeat this to yourself several times per day, and before every nap and bedtime. I promise you'll feel better.
- Practise some self-care – get some early nights, eat easy-to-prepare food, outsource as many tasks as you can, and rope in as much help as you can.

- Consider taking the pressure off yourself. What would happen if you made no effort at all to help your baby sleep? What would happen if you just did whatever you needed to in order to get through this phase? Sometimes, the right decision is to do nothing. You can give yourself permission to do *absolutely nothing* if you lack the capacity for anything else.
- Overhaul your naps. Does your little one need more frequent/less frequent naps?
- What's happened to your bedtime routine? Did you try something that later went belly up? Does it need a rethink? Is it too short/long? Try to have 3-5 predictable and soothing components.[3]
- Use this as an opportunity to rethink anything that isn't working. Is the bath hyping your child up? Be flexible - if it doesn't work for your child, then cut it.

Practical tips to manage nights in a crisis

When you're in the thick of a sleep emergency, it often feels confusing and bleak. The solutions aren't always obvious, and it can be hard to know which strategy to pick. Let me simplify this as much as possible. There are actually only four basic strategies open to you at this point:

1. Change your bedtime
2. Change the person who responds to your child
3. Change the location of your child's sleep
4. Change the response your child gets at night

Of course, within all those changes, there are numerous different options, but I'm assuming you're very tired, and do not have the energy or headspace to sift through them. Let's start with the deal-breakers.

The deal-breakers

The first thing to acknowledge is that there will be things that you have no intention of changing. They are too hard, too important, too meaningful, or just plain impossible. That's okay. Write them down. Maybe you will not, in any circumstance, bed-share. Perhaps you refuse to stop breastfeeding. Or do you have strong feelings about some aspect of your child's bedtime that you are unwilling to compromise on? Anything that you consider a deal-breaker is now officially off the table. We all have different deal-breakers, and yours are important and meaningful. There is almost no circumstance when your deal-breaker will mean you cannot improve your child's sleep and your sleep crisis. The other aspect to remember is that your co-parent may have a different deal-breaker. Discuss this issue, as you may not have realised that both of you value different things. Whatever is left are the aspects you are mutually willing to be flexible with.

Remember, I don't know what your deal-breakers are, so when you read through the suggestions that follow, if any of them would contradict the things that you have decided are important to you, just skip that suggestion and go on to the next one.

Finally, note that most of these suggestions will be suitable for babies over six months. While you may be able to utilise some of these techniques for a younger baby, please bear in mind that babies under six months should be in the same room as their parents during sleep.[4]

1. Change your bedtime

Your bedtime routine is important. It needs to be a time of winding down ready for bed, an opportunity to mark the change in pace of the day, and the shift from wakefulness to sleep. Your child needs to feel safe, secure, loved and responded to in this period. However, if there are elements of your bedtime routine that are not working for your family as a whole, it's okay to change the order, or the elements, of the bedtime. So long as your child still feels safe, secure, loved and responded to, you can, within reason, make changes to it. Think of your bedtime routine as a tower of building blocks. Each block is important and significant. The order, however, is not necessarily as significant. Rather than remove something important from your child's routine, why not just rearrange the sequence? This can feel like a manageable and achievable first step for many people. For example:

Eleni had always breastfed Rosa to sleep. But she was returning to her job, which she loved, and it entailed working nights. She was concerned that if Rosa did not learn to find comfort in other ways to fall asleep, then she would find Eleni's return to work more stressful than it needed to be. Instead of eliminating breastfeeding, as she had initially thought of doing, I suggested she simply move the breastfeed to before the bath. Eleni then held Rosa close to fall asleep instead of feeding her. This opened up options for other people to be able to help Rosa settle down for sleep.

Another way of changing the bedtime routine is to alter the timings of it. This often works well in combination with trying something new. If you try to change something that your child has come to expect, they may find this really hard. But if you capitalise on their natural tiredness, you may find it is a lot easier than you thought.[5,6] For example:

Olly settled for sleep fastest when being rocked by his father, Gus. However, the process often took about an hour, and Gus was getting pretty tired and sore! Gus was worried that if Olly was not rocked to sleep he would cry excessively. In this case, putting Olly to bed half an hour later meant that he was really tired, and when Gus held him still instead of rocking, Olly fell asleep relatively quickly, and without crying.

One more area to think about is the logistics of bedtime: how many components, how much time it takes, the transitions between activities, and the location of the bedtime routine.

If the bedtime routine contains too many elements, it can end up taking too long, and losing focus.[7,8] You can end up with a routine that actually allows your child to get a second lease of life! You'll need to experiment with this to find your magic number and type of activities. Too few elements and your child may not have enough opportunity to calm down. Too many and it becomes more like playtime. Often 3-5 distinct activities work well, but play around.

The bedtime routine should also not take too long. I often suggest that bedtime is like an express train to 'sleepytown'. If the train makes too many stops and takes too long, it can end up taking too long to arrive at the destination. If it is too fast, your child may be hurtled towards sleepytown too fast, not allowing them time to calm down first. How long your bedtime routine should take depends a lot on your child's age and personality. In general, allow for about five minutes per month of age, up to a maximum of 30-40 minutes in total. This does not include the time it takes your child to fall asleep once the lights are out, so the entire bedtime routine from start to asleep should be no more than an hour, allowing for 15-20 minutes to fall asleep.[9]

Sometimes it feels like it is a lot to expect of a child to have them calm down from a fun day in just under an hour. You may find it useful to have a distinct change in pace of the day about 30-60 minutes before you expect your bedtime routine to start. Dim the lights, lower your voice, change the activities, and make a distinct wind-down period with quieter toys and play, soft music or meditations, no screens, and gentle handling.

The activities and their location are also really important. You want to have a natural flow of activities – so if having bathtime too late makes for a tired, cranky child, then have this earlier. If your child has no patience for books last thing before lights out, then have them first of all. If your little one doesn't feed well until they are very sleepy, then you may want to wait until later to feed them. I offer no rules in general, just suggestions that if something isn't working for you or your child, change it in response to your child's natural zones of regulation.[10] One thing to bear in mind is that if bedtime has started, you'll probably find it helpful to remain in the bedroom environment – whether this is your bedroom or your child's. If you find that you and your child end up coming back to the living area, it can send a confusing message about what to expect.

It can be difficult to explain to a very young pre-verbal child that their bedtime routine is about to change. One way that I often suggest is to create a bespoke bedtime book. You simply take photographs of your child at every distinct stage of their bedtime routine – perhaps their pre-bedtime snack or drink, their bath, brushing teeth, having a massage, reading stories and so on. You then print the pictures out into a makeshift 'book'. This becomes your child's illustrated how-to-go-to-sleep guide, personalised for them.

I often suggest that you vary which parent is in the photo, so that your child does not associate 'bedtime' with one particular parent. This is also a good way of introducing your child to the concept that both parents are involved at bedtime.[11]

2. Change the person who responds to your child

The crux of your problem may be that one parent is bearing the brunt of the sleep fragmentation. This may be because of working patterns, the need to breastfeed to sleep, or simply habit. Whatever it is, you may decide that the best option is to switch parents. However, there are numerous ways of involving your co-parent. You could tag-team, take shifts, offer respite, or alternate. You could even consider family or hired help if the situation is desperate and this is an option for you, as people such as doulas have been found to be supportive and improve parenting confidence.[12]

For more than one child, tag-teaming is often a practical option for families, with each parent attending one child. Or you may decide that one parent will do the first part of bedtime, and the second parent will finish off. Working as a team will help stop either of you feeling overwhelmed or under-appreciated.

Taking shifts is another practical option for some families. They may decide that whoever is working the next day will attend to every wake-up before say, midnight. Then every wake up after midnight will be responded to by the parent at home the next day. If you both work, you may each have a natural preference for which side of midnight is more useful to you, or you may need to take turns to get the second stretch of sleep. Another option is that the parent who got the midnight–6am stretch then allows the first shift parent to have an hour or two of sleep first thing in the morning. Or you may allocate this by whoever is most able to get an early night. There is no point after all in taking the second shift if you are unlikely to sleep until midnight anyway.

If things have really come to a head, then the most sleep-deprived parent may need 1–3 nights of respite sleep. There are many things that you might need to consider if you do this. For example – is your child breastfed? If so, then is this age-appropriate? Will you need to express to maintain supply and prevent discomfort? What will you do if your child wakes and is genuinely hungry? Will you offer some limited night feeds but allow your partner to settle your little one after the feed? Will they have expressed milk in a bottle? Remember that you can leave the door open. You can have 1–3 nights of respite, and then return to whatever you were doing before – this is not all or nothing. See the chapter on night feeds for more ideas on how to reduce night feeds.

Finally, you could alternate which parent goes in to respond to night waking. From experience, this strategy can get a little old for some families. The 'your turn', 'my turn' approach can be disruptive for your child, and also doesn't work if one parent is a very heavy sleeper. But if this appeals to you – by all means give it a try.

If you are keen to introduce your child to the idea that more than one parent can be involved with bedtime or helping them fall asleep, then you could overlap for a while. To do this, consider something along the lines of:

- The usual parent does the entire bedtime routine, with the co-parent a passive partner in the background
- The usual parent does the entire bedtime, but the co-parent could do one activity – such as the story. The child remains in the lap or arms of the usual parent throughout
- The usual parent does the beginning part of the bedtime, while the co-parent reads the story with their child on their lap. The usual parent finishes off
- The co-parent completes most of the bedtime, with the usual parent finishing off
- The co-parent does the entire bedtime, with the usual parent a passive partner in the background

Exactly how you work this is entirely up to you – this is just an idea. You may need to introduce additional steps, or spend longer on certain steps, as your child adjusts.

3. Change the location of your child's sleep

This is another quite practical strategy if the location of sleep is the area that is specifically causing stress. First, you'll need to think about where your child falls asleep. Be very specific. Is it a chest? A shoulder? Your arms? On the breast? In your bed? Making one small change to this can be really helpful to make sleep feel more sustainable again. Doing something constructive can feel like a positive step forward to make nights feel more manageable.[13] Could your child fall asleep in your arms instead of at the breast? Or if they usually fall asleep upright, over your shoulder, could you hold them horizontally in arms instead? If they are currently in your bed, could you move to a floor bed? You may find that you end up making these changes in a small step-wise fashion, for example:

1. Falling asleep at the breast
2. Feeding earlier in the routine, then falling asleep upright in arms (parent standing)
3. Falling asleep horizontally in arms (parent standing)
4. Falling asleep horizontally in arms (parent sitting)
5. Falling asleep lying on mattress on floor with parent lying right beside
6. Falling asleep in cot, with parent lying beside

I would suggest that you decide the steps, and let your child decide how quickly to progress through the steps.

4. Change the response your child gets at night

Last of all, you could alter what response your child gets in the night. There are four main ways of altering the response – either add in sleep cues, overlap new cues, delay the usual response, or remove the usual response.

If you decide to add in extra sleep cues, you'll probably discover that this is not enough by itself as a strategy. I have met many frustrated parents who read that a comforter would help their child to settle, only to find that their child threw their bunny across the room, and sleep was still elusive. Nevertheless, it's still a useful tool to have in your toolbox. Try sleeping with your child's cot sheet so that it smells of you. I also sometimes suggest sticking photos of loved ones around your child's sleep space – this is more useful with older babies and toddlers. If your child is old enough to recognise people, then they may like to have familiar faces around them.

A more successful strategy is to overlap new sleep cues,[14] which is based on the concept of 'habit stacking'.[15] What you are essentially doing with this is acknowledging that your child's favourite way of falling asleep is highly successful. It may not be sustainable, but it *is* effective. You're going to capitalise on that effectiveness by trying to attach or overlap new cues at the same time. Let's say your child usually prefers to be fed back to sleep. If your child's favourite sleep cue is rocking, or coming in to your bed, or being held, then substitute that whenever you see the word 'feeding'! You'll spend 2–3 weeks (or more) overlapping new cues on to your child's favourite. So instead of just feeding, you'll also pat, shush, and introduce a comfort object. I like to tap in to as many senses as possible, but pay attention to what your child finds soothing. They may not like patting, but like their face being stroked, or their back rubbed. They may not like shushing, but settle faster with deep breathing, or gentle humming, or even white noise.

Then, when you feel ready, instead of allowing your child to fall asleep completely while feeding, stop the feed just a little earlier, but maintain all the other soothing sleep cues. You're aiming for your child to barely notice, and not suddenly wake up. Ideally, your child will remain calm, and not get upset. You will ultimately have your child feeding awake, then having a cuddle in arms, before being placed in their sleep space asleep. You can then move on to holding them until they are calm, but awake, then put them down and continue to shush and pat until they are asleep. You're essentially adding in layers of support, and then slowly peeling off those layers. You can take your time, and go at your child's pace. This is probably the slowest and gentlest way to modify sleep, but you will eventually get to where you want to be.

Another option is to delay the response. I don't mean that you will leave your little one crying! But instead of immediately doing what you usually do to resettle your child, just pause for a moment and procrastinate a little before feeding them. If they are making noises but you do not feel they are upset, then just wait a moment. The French call this 'le pause'. Change their nappy, or give them a cuddle. Instead of bringing them straight to your bed, wait a while to see if they will go back to sleep if you stay with them. Sometimes we assume that this won't happen before we have given it a chance.[16] Another way of doing this is to send your co-parent in, and let them try to resettle for a specified amount of time that you feel comfortable with, or until your little one becomes upset.

Finally, you could remove the expected response – which is probably the fastest, but hardest option. I tend to reserve this option for when there is no other choice. It's really important to acknowledge that sometimes a sleep emergency requires a faster solution. This may be due to a physical or mental health emergency, contextual situation, or family problem. Everyone has a different threshold for what they can cope with. This strategy can be hard, as your little one has come to expect a certain response. While you will still be responsive, change is hard for little people.

I firmly believe that the best way to remove your child's expected response is to provide an alternative that includes as much as reassurance and comfort as they need. Sometimes parents question this – asking whether they will essentially be replacing one unsustainable activity for another equally unsustainable one. I can see why people might think that, but I think of it more as a sideways step in order to achieve a forward goal. In my experience, once you widen the repertoire of activities that your child finds soothing, they begin to accept other ways of falling asleep, which will ultimately give you more options, or allow other people to be involved. For example:

Angie was becoming exhausted from her 14-month-old Harry's waking. He wanted the breast to fall asleep every single time he woke, and while this worked in the early months, it was becoming increasingly unmanageable. Her husband was sleeping on the sofa and they were falling out. Angie decided to cuddle Harry in her bed initially while she set limits on night feeds. She decided she would feed Harry no more than every three hours at night, and then would work towards only feeding him 1-2 times. Harry found this hard for a few nights, but Angie held him close, whispering to him, and rubbing his back.

Georgia was 11 months old and had to be rocked back to sleep several times per night. This was becoming unsustainable, so her parents decided they would hold Georgia still instead of rocking her. The problem remained though that Georgia would often wake up when transferred to her cot. Her parents decided to take Georgia's mattress out of her cot, because it made settling her easier. This way, they could hold her close, but did not need to do the dreaded transfer to the cot. They planned to work towards reassembling the cot once Georgia was waking up less.

Floor beds, bed-sharing and crying in arms

You may need a different approach to helping your child fall asleep if they have become used to a certain sleep trigger. One of my favourite tricks is a floor bed – an idea borrowed from Montessori ideology.[17] This avoids the need to transfer children from arms to cot. This makes a lot of sense if you have just spent time and effort getting your little one to sleep and then they promptly wake up on transfer. Some people will reject this instantly. Maybe your room cannot be made safe and you have a little explorer on your hands. Maybe your children share a room and it isn't practical. It's not a solution that will work for everyone, but it may be an option for some. Indeed, some families like the floor bed so much, they keep it. Some ideas for making it work include:

- Strip the room down to the bare essentials
- Put a single mattress on the floor instead of a cot mattress – this gives you room to lie next to your child

- Put a single mattress on the floor next to your own double or king-size mattress

You can reassemble the mattress once sleep is going better (if you want to), then move on to lying next to the cot on the mattress.

Bed-sharing may be what you're trying to move on from, but it might also be a tool to maximise sleep in a crisis. Perhaps you've never bed-shared, but for the sake of everyone getting the most sleep possible, you might feel you want to consider it. See the section on bed-sharing to make an informed decision about whether this is right and safe for your family. If you're already sharing your bed with your baby, you may want to continue for a little while longer while you night wean, or limit night feeds – you'll probably find it easier than traipsing back and forth to another room.

Finally, your little one may cry during any of these strategies. If you feel you could have a rethink, do things slower, or wait till a better time, then it's okay to pause. If at any time it doesn't feel right, then trust your gut. However, as you found out in the chapter about crying, babies and children cry for many reasons, and while those reasons are always meaningful, not all crying is the same. Crying in the arms of a loving, responsive parent is hugely different from crying alone. If you are in a genuine sleep crisis, and have no choice but to make changes, then sometimes you have to be pragmatic. If you decide on a strategy that involves your little one being held and comforted, then rest assured that you are still being responsive. What I'm not a big fan of is people throwing around the term 'sleep crisis' to justify a less responsive sleep strategy. I have worked with some parents who are in awful situations, and I know full well that sometimes change really is essential. I don't like to hear of crying in arms being put forward as a strategy for babies if there is an alternative, but equally, I don't like to hear of parents feeling terrible that their child cried while being loved and held and soothed when there was simply no choice.

Combining strategies

Of course, in practice you may read through this and decide that you need to work on several areas. I would still urge you to make small, manageable changes. Addressing several things at once can feel overwhelming in the midst of sleep deprivation. Consider doing one change at a time, unless a few seem to group together well. Also, remember that you may need to think of a strategy for feeding and sleeping separately. Since stopping night feeding does not always stop night waking, you may need to work on both of these at the same time. For example:

> *Hannah and Lori were struggling with Wallis's sleep. Wallis was eight months old and waking every 40 minutes all night. After considering all their options, they decided that they would optimise naps, work on sleep hygiene and improve their own emotional and psychological wellbeing with mindfulness and alternate nostril breathing, as well as listening to meditations before sleep times. Since Lori and Hannah were both working part-time and sharing the care of Wallis at home, they decided that they would both be involved at bedtime, and then take turns with who got respite nights, depending on who was working the following day. Hannah was breastfeeding Wallis, and they rearranged the bedtime routine so that Wallis was not falling asleep feeding. To minimise crying, they made bedtime temporarily later, to capitalise on high sleep pressure and an easier time falling asleep, moving it earlier as he adjusted. They also decided to set some reasonable limits on night feeds, reducing the feeds to two feeds at around 11pm and 3am, which they felt was manageable.*

Every family will have their own story of sleep crisis, and the things they need to do in order to feel able to cope again. I urge you to make small changes that you can live with, and that feel in-line with your parenting values and priorities. Decide on your deal-breakers, and respect those boundaries.

The tired parent's summary:

- Everyone has a different level of challenge with sleep. You will find you require a different approach depending on the urgency of your situation.
- Sleep crises are not experienced by everyone. They tend to describe an unsustainable and unmanageable level of sleep deprivation or disruption.

- A sleep crisis needs a different approach to a simple sleep problem, but never needs to involve a non-response or crying alone.
- Sleep crises may be contextual – related to your or your child's health or family circumstances, or an emergency situation.
- During a crisis, you can still choose to tackle problems slowly, and step by step, or you may need a faster strategy.
- Working on underlying causes of sleep crises – whether these are psychological, physical, or behavioural – will usually be the best solution.
- Simplifying sleep strategies down to four basic themes can help you to feel less overwhelmed by options.
- Even in a crisis, you do not need to do anything you feel uncomfortable with. Decide on your deal-breakers and work with your co-parent to respect and honour their deal-breakers too.
- Sometimes simple changes to timings, bedtime routine and other small adaptations can be a game-changer for sleep. Don't lose hope!

Chapter twelve

Situational sleep stress

→ There are some moments when sleep fragmentation comes into sharp focus because of the context. It may be that you were coping before, but a change has either worsened your little one's sleep, or you have fewer reserves to cope with it. You might just be more anxious about sleep because of the context. I can't possibly know your situation, but I hope you can find what you're looking for among some of these common scenarios.

Returning to work

This can be time of immense personal inner conflict and confusion. It can also put pressure on your sleep situation. I am frequently contacted by parents who are imminently returning to work, and are worried that they will not be able to cope with the demands of their job on the back of poor sleep. There are several elements to unpick:

- Will it *really* be harder when you go back to work?
- Are there some confusing and anxiety-provoking emotions getting entangled with sleep?
- Do you feel forced back to the workplace, and resent having to work on sleep because of a job you do not want to return to?
- Do you feel guilty because you are actually really looking forward to your return to work?
- Are you anxious about leaving your baby?
- Will your job ever take you away overnight?
- Do you work night shifts?
- Are you anxious about childcare, or what your baby will eat and drink while you are away from them?

There are three main themes that I encounter from parents: a feeling that work will be hard to cope with if you aren't sleeping well, complex emotions, and how your baby will sleep without you present.

Firstly, you may be stressed about sleep because you are anxious that work will be unmanageable on your current sleep. I do not know what job you do, but there may be more to unpick here than you think. Working away from the home environment requires a mental shift, and your concern may be that if you are fatigued, you will not be able to perform your job well. I think this is a really rational concern. However, you may actually find that being in a new environment, with adult company, the ability to have a break, and some other tasks to focus your mind on may be easier than you fear. It is said that a change is as good as a rest – many parents tell me that their fears were unfounded, and that they returned to work, surrounded by colleagues and hot coffee, and enjoyed the stimulation of work and adult conversation. Being at home while you are very tired can actually feel even more exhausting. I used to joke that working in neonatal intensive care, caring for up to 40 families with complex needs, was far easier than looking after my then two-year-old. However, it is not always true that work is easier. I have found that the vast majority of parents find parenting to be the most challenging (and rewarding) job of all, and find work to be *less* strenuous than being at home, but I have run into a few exceptions. I once worked with an academic whose job was to peer review journal articles. She was falling asleep at her desk. Of course, there are many factors to consider, but I would urge you to think long and hard before deciding that you need to change your sleep situation due to your impending return to work. It may not be as bad as you think.

Very often a parent will have mixed feelings about returning to work. I don't know if you adore your job, or simply have to work for financial reasons. Do you need to remain in the workplace for career prospects even though there is very little financial gain? I appreciate the wide variety of situations you may find yourself in. There is sometimes a combination of excitement and anxiety. It's very important to have someone with whom you can be honest about your feelings and emotions. Whatever you're feeling is valid, and probably completely normal and understandable. If you feel very conflicted or unhappy, this may be something that you would benefit from discussing with a psychotherapist with experience in this area. In the meantime, please remember your self-care: eat and drink well, get plenty of exercise, practise some mindfulness or guided relaxation, and talk to friends and family. Finally, I would encourage you to think about your options to improve your work-life balance. I appreciate that not all of these strategies will be applicable to everyone, so pick and choose the ones that might work for you:

- Is there a possibility of you and your partner both working part-time so that you can share the care of your child(ren) without needing any formal childcare? You may find that the reduction in pay works out to be more cost-effective than paid childcare.
- Can you work part-time, or at least start off part-time and work up to more hours?
- Can you work longer hours on fewer days per week?
- Could you work shorter hours on more days per week?
- Is there a possibility of finishing early every day and finishing off work from home after your child has gone to bed?
- Could you work from home?
- Can you ask a family member to care for your child if that would be easier or more affordable – thereby reducing the hours you need to work?
- If you are still breastfeeding, have you considered the following options:
  - Have your childcare close to your workplace so you can visit your baby to breastfeed during the working day
  - Have your nanny bring your baby into work so that you can

breastfeed them
- Have you asked your employer where you can express and store your breastmilk? You are protected by law to be able to do this
- If your baby will be older than about 6-8 months, you may find that they take very well to solids and don't actually need as much milk in the day
- Can you use your annual leave to extend your parental leave?

It's worth exploring all your options, so that you know you have made a fully informed decision. Many people return to work after having children, and the truth is that once you find the right childcare that you are happy with, and have allowed yourself a settling back in period, it does get easier. Be kind to yourself.

Finally, your concerns about sleep and work may be more related to how your baby will manage to fall asleep without you. If your baby has been dependent on you feeding them to sleep for naps and bedtime, you may be wondering how they will fall asleep without you. Or if you are planning to work away from home overnight, either because your job requires you to be away for several days at a time, or you work night shifts, you may also have some questions. I have a few suggestions if this is your situation:

- Can you use some of the gentle strategies to help your baby learn that that there are other ways of falling asleep?
- If the thought of changing how your baby falls asleep makes you sad or stressed, you could consider making a positive choice to not change anything. Your baby will learn that when you are around, they can fall asleep one way, and when you're not around, they will have another attentive caregiver help them fall asleep.
- Can you delay your first night shift until you have been back at work for several weeks, to allow you both time to adjust?
- Find out from your place of work when your first overnight trip will be.
- Is taking your baby, along with a family member, on overnight trips an option?

Whatever your situation, you almost always have options – even if your only choice is to either change the way your little one falls asleep or do nothing. It's still a choice, and it's yours to make.

Expecting another baby

I have lost count of the number of parents who get in touch because they are worried about sleep in the context of expecting baby number two, or three, or more. I find most parents fall in to one of two categories:

1. You had a difficult sleep experience with your eldest or previous child, and while they now sleep well, you want to spare yourself the headache of going through that again
2. Your older child still does not sleep well, is still breastfeeding at night or is bed-sharing, and you are wondering how you will manage this with a new baby as well

1. Previous difficult experience

Firstly, I'm so sorry that you found sleep stressful before. I hesitate to use the word 'trauma', but I honestly feel that the stress and anxiety of a previous sleep crisis can be intense. Expecting another baby can cause some of these past or buried feelings to bubble to the surface. You may feel like you are worried about a potential problem before it is even upon you. If I was with you, the first thing I would want to do is give you a hug. Of course, that's not very professional, and fundamentally, I am not there, so you'll have to accept a virtual hug.

The second thing I would do is validate your experience. Everyone has a different sleep journey and threshold for finding a situation unmanageable. Nobody has the right to judge whether you were right to find your experience stressful. So I acknowledge the stress and strain that your sleep situation caused.

Thirdly, I would want to reassure you that no two babies are the same. Just because you had a difficult experience last time does not mean the same thing will happen again. Nobody can promise that it will be the exact opposite either, but I urge you not to project the expectation that you will re-experience a sleep crisis with this new baby.

Next, I would want to help you to manage your own emotional health and wellbeing. Since we know that managing and overcoming prenatal stress can improve the sleep of the unborn child, it makes a lot of sense for you to find ways of combating stress and mental and emotional health. If you feel you need more support than basic self-care, then I urge you to speak to your healthcare professional or a psychotherapist/

counsellor who can help you to work past these unhelpful feelings.

Finally, take some positive steps. Go back to the chapters on normal infant sleep, and how to optimise sleep in infants, and make sure that your expectations, and your plan for this baby, are realistic. Remember, sometimes we have a tendency to remember the stand-out negative moments. Your newborn baby will definitely sleep erratically, wake frequently, and need to be supported to sleep – but none of these sleep features means that they will have the same sleep experience as your previous child.

2. Your older child still doesn't sleep well

You may be concerned about your older child or children not sleeping well for many reasons. The most common reasons I encounter are either that parents are concerned about further sleep deprivation when they are already exhausted, or that they are worried about the practicalities of tandem breastfeeding or having more than one child potentially in bed. Let's cover these main issues separately.

If you are primarily concerned about compounded sleep deprivation, then you could take some steps to try to improve your older child's sleep. These might include moving them out of your bed, reducing night feeds, or improving the way they fall asleep at bedtime. It might even be a combination of all three! Go back to the chapters on addressing a sleep crisis, as well as how to optimise sleep. The following strategies might be helpful:

- Work on naps – most 18–30-month-old children still need one nap per day
- Do you have a soothing, gentle bedtime routine?
- Does your child resist bedtime? If so, are they going to bed too early? Or are they perhaps overtired? You may need to review your timings if bedtime is the sticking point.
- Ensure your toddler or preschooler has plenty of exercise and healthy food, and try to minimise screen time in the two hours before a nap or bedtime
- Try to have at least 10 minutes of completely focused, undistracted time every day with your older child. I know you probably spend vastly more time than this with your child, but I'm talking about really focused, intense, child-led, one-to-one time. Ten minutes of playing like this is immensely beneficial. I often say that this type of

play fills up a child's 'love tank'. The more you fill up their love tank, the less likely they are to whine and play up at bedtime due to feeling disconnected.

- Have you considered a floor bed next to your bed to move your child away from bed-sharing? This can be a good bridge to getting them to sleep in their own bed
- How do you feel about tandem feeding if you are still breastfeeding? Some people are open to the idea, while others are desperate to stop feeding their older child. It is a very personal decision. I strongly suggest you reach out to a breastfeeding counsellor or IBCLC for more support with this.

You do not have to work on all these areas at the same time. Just pick the most manageable strategies from this list and work consistently on them.

The practicalities of having two children with similar yet different needs may also be on your mind. It is perfectly possible to breastfeed a newborn and a toddler.[1] While many toddlers and preschoolers wean during pregnancy, either because milk supply drops, or they don't like the change in taste, some hang in there. If you are lactating, remember it is your body and you get to say how it is used, by whom, and for how long. You have options. Please call for specialist breastfeeding support if you need more information about these issues.

Secondly, if your little one is in your bed, then you may have some questions about the practicalities of this. It is not safe for an infant and older child to sleep side by side. A responsive, attentive adult needs to be beside a newborn, or the newborn needs to be in their own sleep space. Review the information about safe sleep in the normal infant sleep chapter, and check whether there are any reasons why you should definitely not bed-share. Otherwise, make a plan for how you will manage once the new baby arrives. Some options are as follows:

- Will the new baby go in a side-car crib while your older child stays in your bed?
- Will you start to transition your older child to a floor bed in your room, then on to their own bed?
- Do you want to plan to have your older child on one side of you, and the new baby on your other side?

Your decisions about where your children will sleep are very personal, and also involve your partner if you have one. Will there be room for everyone to sleep where they want to sleep? And will this be safe, practical and comfortable? These are decisions that only you, with your knowledge of your home, bed, children, partner and self, can decide.

Teething

Typing 'teething' into Google yields over 20 million hits. It's a big topic in parenting. It's often blamed for a multitude of sleep problems.

The actual mechanisms of teething are not well understood,[2] but it is thought that hormones are responsible for skin cell death in the gum. This cellular death causes the gums to break apart and allows space for the erupting tooth below the gum-line. The words people use for teething are often unhelpful, and lead us to attribute more pain to teething than is probably the reality. We talk about 'cutting' teeth, for example, but the teeth do not physically slice the gums.

When do teeth first appear?

There is huge variability with the eruption of teeth. Some babies get their first tooth at just a few weeks, or they are even present from birth,[3] while other babies' first birthdays come and go long before the first pearly white. Teeth usually erupt in pairs, and on average, the tooth eruption process is as follows:

1. The two lower central incisors – around six months
2. The two upper central incisors – around eight months
3. The two lateral upper and lower incisors – around 10 months
4. The first four molars – around 14 months
5. The four canines – around 18 months
6. The second four molars – between 2-3 years

Many people think a baby is teething at around three months. This is usually due to the fact that a baby will typically start to drool, and also be able to start getting their hand accurately to their mouth and chewing it. Often people put these two signs together and assume that teeth are to blame, when this is actually a normal developmental stage.

The process of teething is often felt to be long, arduous and protracted. Unsettled behaviour, fussing and unexplained sleep disturbance are often unfairly blamed on teething, when in actual fact they are more likely to be caused by something else.

What is teething blamed for?

Over the centuries, teething has been blamed for all manner of evils, from diarrhoea and nappy/diaper rash, to intractable pain and even death. In fact, in 1842, records show that in nearly 5 percent of all infant deaths, teething was named as the cause, and it apparently caused 7 percent of all deaths in 1–3-year-olds. Of course, now we know better, but certainly, anxiety about teething is not a new phenomenon.

Nowadays, it is more likely that people will blame teething for any unexplained period of fussing or sleep disturbance. It is important to state that the actual process of dentition usually takes about 3–6 days. That's it. This is really important, because unexplained cranky behaviour, fussing, sleep disturbance and illness that lasts longer than this is very likely to be caused by something else.

The truth is that babies are nearly always going through one developmental stage or another. If it's not a gross or fine motor developmental learning curve, it's social awareness. If it's not learning to babble, it's learning to sit up, or crawl. If it's not separation anxiety, it's probably mastering some complex hand-eye coordination task. So if a baby seems to be cranky or fussy for several weeks, it's more likely to be caused by back-to-back developmental phases, rather than a tooth – which usually causes quite a distinct, short phase of obvious fuss.

This is important to know, for many reasons, but one is unnecessary medication. You see, if parents attribute long drawn-out phases of fussing to teething, their very reasonable assumption is that teething is a long, protracted, painful process. What parent wants their child to be in pain for days or weeks on end? But the problem is that a) pain relief won't help if it's a developmental phase, b) unnecessary pain relief could be harmful,[4] and c) it leads parents to believe that their child is really suffering from teething pain which is intractable and not resolvable with simple analgesia. This serves to reinforce the belief that teething is a very painful process. It also potentially means that a child will be given pain relief at the first onset of fussy behaviour – which could be around four months, only for the first tooth to not arrive until eight or nine months. That's five months of unnecessary medication, and a reinforced belief that teeth take months to emerge and are very painful.

- **Gas/wind** There is no evidence that teething causes this. It is more likely to be due to something the baby ate. Don't forget, babies are often getting teeth around the same time they are trying lots of new foods. It could just be that one of them has caused their system to react with more gas than usual.

- **Fever** While teething is an inflammatory process, it will not cause a significant fever. A very low-grade fever of up to about 37.9°C (100.2°F) may be caused by teething,[5] if there are other obvious signs as well, but a fever higher than this is almost certainly caused by an illness, such as a virus.

- **Coughs, runny nose and colds** There is no evidence that teething causes a viral illness such as a cold or cough. It doesn't really make a lot of physiological sense. Teething is an inflammatory process, so it is plausible that the immune system is under more strain than usual, but even that is a stretch. What is more likely is that babies of the age to start teething are more exposed to new environments, germs and new people who are spreading coughs and colds. Approximately 10 colds per year is entirely normal for young children – which can feel almost endless during the winter months. Babies often start day care or nursery around the time they start teething, so it is likely that this is a coincidence.

- **Diarrhoea** It is highly improbable that teething causes diarrhoea. Lots of parents anecdotally report that their baby has a 'vinegar' smelling nappy around the time of teething, but true diarrhoea (very loose, runny, watery, foul-smelling stool) is not likely to be caused by teething. It is far more likely that the baby has touched something or been exposed to a bug that has upset their tummy. Don't forget, around the time babies start teething, they are also crawling around, putting everything in their mouth, touching the dog's rear end, putting other children's chewed toys in their mouths – you get the picture!

- **Nappy/diaper rash** Again, this is a common young childhood complaint. While lots of parents report some nappy rash around the time of teething, it is just as likely to be caused by something their little one ate that has caused a particularly offensive stool. If your baby has had a 'vinegar poo' then it is possible that the skin may be more irritated than usual, but a significant nappy/diaper rash should not just be attributed to teething, in case it is a fungal or bacterial rash that needs medical attention.

So, what can teething cause?

So, now you know what teething probably *doesn't* cause, you'll most likely want to know what it *does* cause. Here we go:

- **Pain** Teething causes inflammation and swelling. This can be painful, no denying it. Nobody wants their little one to be in pain. Actually, some babies don't seem to be bothered by teething at all. And others will really let you know about it. In fact, both my own two children were completely different. One shouted and screeched for three days, while the other just woke up and there it was – we knew nothing about its impending arrival. It is not uncommon for parents to experience a totally different reaction from different children. I can only put this down to differences in pain perception, different inflammatory responses, and different anatomy.
- **Sleep problems** Teething can cause a variety of problems with sleep. Common symptoms include:
  - More frequent breastfeeding (the action of breastfeeding soothes the pressure in the jaw and mouth)
  - Drooling
  - Chewing on lots of hard objects – including knuckles, wooden toys, feet, utensils and any other hard object they can lay their hands on
  - Reluctance to eat
  - Pulling at their ears
  - Bright red cheeks

These symptoms are actually quite specific, and focused around the jaw and mouth itself. It should be fairly obvious when a child is teething – it will be 3–5 days of gnawing and chewing, and possible fussing.

So, does this affect sleep? Well, it may do. It is important to note that teething does not always seem to cause a baby any trouble. But other babies seem to have trouble with teething for a few possible reasons:

1. There are fewer distractions in the night-time. In the day, a baby may be more easily pacified with a toy, a change of scene, or a cuddle. At night, it is dark, quiet, and there is less stimulation. As distraction is a well-known form of pain relief, it makes total sense that nights would be worse than days.

2. Babies usually lie down to sleep. In the daytime, when they are upright, there is less blood flow to the head. Lying down may increase the pressure in the head. This is also true of any sinus-related pain – it is always better once you are standing upright, due to gravity.
3. Fatigued babies may be more cranky and irritable. So, the link between tiredness, poor sleep and teething may be closely related.

Is there anything you can do about teething?

Many parents want to know what to do about teething. Any pharmaceutical shelf will have a wide array of gels, powders, and granules to rub on the gums to ease teething pain. Some good general advice is that if you are not sure if your baby is unwell, or teething, you should get them seen by a doctor. For example: a baby with a fever, who is reluctant to feed, and pulling their ears may have an ear infection, rather than an imminent new tooth. Rubbing teething gel on their gums will do nothing to address the underlying condition.

If you are certain that this is new behaviour, specific to teething, then you could certainly try a teething gel or homeopathic remedy. But I would urge you to not use these for more than a few days. If your baby is still upset after this, it is more likely to be something else.

There are many parents who feel more comfortable trying non-pharmacological remedies. Some simple ones include:

- Putting a clean flannel/washcloth in a plastic bag and freezing it. Let it thaw a little before giving it to the baby – frozen flannels can stick painfully to lips
- Offer cold, hard, watery foods to chew – such as cucumber, melon and frozen banana (again – thaw a little first)
- Make a 'momsicle' or 'booby lolly' – use expressed breastmilk (or formula) to make a milk popsicle that your baby can suck

Some people want to try Baltic amber teething necklaces or bracelets. The theory is that the amber is warmed against the skin and slowly releases pain-relieving and anti-inflammatory properties to ease teething pain. *There is no evidence to back this up.* The problems with this strategy are:

- It feeds into the idea that teething is a long drawn-out process
- They pose a choking risk
- They are a strangulation hazard

Instead:

- Try teething chew toys that are specifically designed for teething babies. Some can be chilled first
- Consider naps in a baby carrier to have your baby upright
- Try to prioritise sleep as much as possible, using any means necessary – it will prevent crankiness. You may need to accept some flexibility on sleep location during this acute phase
- Promote a stress-free environment. Since stress can cause inflammation, try to optimise a calming atmosphere. This is also good for bonding and is more conducive to sleep!

Illness

When little ones are unwell, it is of course expected that they will need more help and have more disturbed sleep. It is also entirely appropriate to give that extra help and support to an unwell child. Most people have no problem with this. Of course, it is exhausting and worrying when a child is ill, but the vast majority of parents would never dream of denying their child extra comfort when they are not feeling well. The tricky part is figuring out when the illness has passed, and how to get back on track after illness.

My experience as a nurse has taught me that when children and babies are mildly unwell, they may sleep far *less* than usual, be cranky and irritable, go off solid food, prefer milk feeds, and need more cuddles and comfort. When children are more unwell, including with a high fever, they tend to be much quieter, sleep a lot more than usual, and eat nothing at all. I always worried far more about the quiet children than the noisy ones. Discomforts such as blocked or runny nose, cough, fever, headache and joint pain may make your child feel generally unwell and miserable. With the exception of cough, which is pretty self-explanatory, it is highly unlikely that your child can adequately describe these symptoms in any meaningful way. You are stuck with having to guess what the problem is.

Night feeds during illness

You may have been reducing night feeds gently when your child became unwell, only to find that night feeds increase during illness. Most children will want and need more feeds at night when they are unwell because

> **" Part of being responsive is knowing when you need to scale up and when it's okay to scale back. "**

they are comforting, and because they may be thirstier. If your child's primary comfort measure is feeding, then it is likely that you will revert to your child's previous pattern of frequent night feeds. All is not lost, I promise! Part of being responsive is knowing when you need to scale up and when it's okay to scale back.

Having a fever often causes children to sweat more, and therefore become a little dehydrated. If your child has a blocked nose it will cause them to mouth breathe, which will lead to a dry mouth. Fever and sweating, and mouth breathing, will probably lead to an increase in night feeds or drinks.

Many people think that if their child's appetite has diminished, that they will feed more in the night to compensate. There may be some truth in this if a baby has gone off their solid food – they may want more milk feeds to compensate. However, if the child has gone off all feeds, then waking in the night is very unlikely to be caused by hunger – we do not suddenly recover our appetite in the middle of the night when unwell. What is more likely is that the child has a dry mouth or is feeling thirsty due to fever and sweating.

How to know the illness has passed

This may sound like an obvious point – after all, surely you would know that an illness has passed? But actually, children are constantly developing – so a cold can be fading out just as a major developmental phase is beginning. Or croup can strike right on the back of a new tooth, followed by learning to crawl. Life is not neatly and clearly demarcated by events interspersed by quiet periods of calm – sometimes they blur and merge into each other. So there are some clues you can look for to try to figure out if your child's illness has passed or if you are still in the thick of it:

- **Fever** Absence of fever is a pretty good clue that your child is over the worst of their illness, although children do not always have a noticeable fever with a very mild cough and cold.
- **Appetite** Most children go off food during acute illness, and becoming interested in food again is a very good clue that they feel better.
- **Energy levels** Many babies and children will become listless, quiet, or sleepier. They often lose interest in playing and just want to be

cuddled more. Resuming interest in play and toys is a pretty good sign you're over the worst of it, although children can be incredibly stoical. Sometimes they will play while their fever is down, and then stop playing when it spikes again. I remember working on paediatric wards and knowing instinctively when a particular child needed their temperature taking again due to the change in their energy levels.

- **Behaviour** It is an unusual child who patiently tolerates being unwell. The vast majority of babies and children are cranky, miserable, cry more and fuss during illness. Being alert to this behaviour fading out can help you figure out whether you're over the illness. As I said before, children's behaviour will often mirror fluctuations in fever, so what you're looking for is a return to less cranky behaviour that is sustained over at least 12 hours. Sometimes a fever can come and go but get less frequent.

My very wise grandmother (a Dutch nurse, born in the 1920s) passed on a nugget of advice to my own mother, which is that you should observe 24 hours of wellness and absence of fever before declaring an illness over. It is excellent advice, and I share it with you in the hope that it helps you in your child's illness management.

When you think the illness has passed, you'll probably find it easiest to go back to basics:

- Be child-led – observe what your child needs. They may need more or less sleep in the period immediately following illness. Be flexible and be prepared to scale up or down the number of sleep opportunities you provide.
- Try to resume your usual routines for before sleep. These often go out of the window during illness, so pick them back up again and be patient.
- If you were already trying to improve sleep when this happened, you'll need to accept that these backward steps are normal and part of the overall progress. Go back to the nearest step to your current situation. It's a classic three-steps-forward-four-steps-back situation. Progress is almost never consistently linear, and that's okay.
- Get plenty of exercise, fresh air, and good nutrition.

Illness is an almost inevitable part of childhood, and it is highly likely that you will have to deal with a setback caused by illness if you are working on sleep. There is no magic or easy way to prevent sleep setbacks – all you can do is continue to provide your gentle, consistent, comforting care, and accept that progress will be up and down.

Moving home

Often, as a family expands, a house move is an inevitable next step. Let's face it, there is almost never a good time to schedule a house move – it is right up in the top 10 most stressful things to do (sorry!). Perhaps you're worried about your child's sleep being disrupted by your house move, or maybe you're wondering whether you should try to optimise your child's sleep before the move, or delay it until after you've moved.

If you're about to pack up and move home, I think it is realistic to say that this is an unsettling time for everyone in the household. If you're feeling anxious about it, chances are your little one may find it unsettling too. I'm sure you will already be doing plenty to minimise the stress, but here are a few ideas from a serial mover (I grew up in a military family and have been through this well over 30 times):

- Make sure you pack a box or suitcase with your essential items: toys, familiar objects and at least three days' worth of clothes for everyone. Pack sanitary items nearby, because isn't it always the case that a period arrives at the exact moment when you're least prepared? Stress can make a menstrual cycle go haywire, so it may be erratic and unexpected.
- Plan to set up your sleep space first, with familiar sleep clothes and bedding for you and your child(ren).
- If you can afford to, hire a removal company who can also pack for you as well. It is often not much more to have them pack as well as lift and shift the heavy boxes. It only takes 48 hours and you can live in relative normality for as long as possible without endless evenings packing up. Money well spent...
- Enlist as many people to help as possible.
- Consider delegating the actual house move day to someone, while you escape the madness with your child and rest somewhere till the worst is over!
- Buy or make meals for the freezer, so that you don't actually have to cook for several days after the move.
- When you move in, walk your little one through the house in your

arms, and show them where all the rooms are.

- Place photos of familiar people around the walls of your child's room or sleep space.
- Try if you can to maintain familiar routines, stories, and systems.

It is probably also realistic to accept a certain level of chaos in the sleep department for a few days before and after your move. Don't forget, your little one's world is smaller than yours. They have less perspective and life experience. For them, their usual familiar space is turned upside down by moving. Be patient and kind to yourself and your child.

Finally, I would definitely suggest waiting until you've been in your new home for a couple of weeks at least, unpacked the sleep spaces, and feel calmer. A certain amount of disruption is absolutely to be expected, so don't panic if the sleep deteriorates. You may find it improves spontaneously when things settle down, but if not, at least you won't be hunting desperately through packing materials to find the blackout blind.

Family upheaval

I can't possibly know what this phrase means to you. It might mean a distressing event, a separation, or a family crisis. Whatever it is, if you identify with this, I'm so sorry for the stress that your family is under. I have no magic or quick answers for you, but I do have some suggestions. Firstly, whoever is your child's usual caregiver is their rock, their fortress, their safe space and their comfort. Do everything in your power to safeguard the sanctuary of that relationship. If your child will be cared for by others, then if you can, try to ensure that the person is familiar. When our youngest daughter was diagnosed with cancer, our eldest was cared for by a combination of my husband, grandparents, and very close friends. The playdates were a novelty at first, but after a while they got old. She longed for the safety and familiarity of her mum. So while I do not know your unique circumstances, I too have known upheaval, drama and crisis. Some strategies that might help:

- Keep a going-away bag nearby, with familiar and comforting objects.
- Leave an article of clothing that smells like the missed parent.
- Arrange the time apart so that it is not excessive.
- If you are breastfeeding, and in the middle of a separation, get support

and legal advice from someone who understands the breastfeeding relationship and attachment.

- Make a bespoke bedtime book – take photos of your child in different settings at distinct stages of their bedtime routine and use this as a way of preparing them for a different location or home.
- Allow and invite your child to ask questions. If you do not allow a verbal child to ask questions, they may invent a more frightening reality in their head.
- Try as far as possible to have similar or even identical routines, timings and stories to reassure your child in different settings.

If you are struggling with a major turbulence, I cannot urge you enough to ensure that you practise self-care and also ask for help if you need more support. I hope things get easier for you.

Travelling and going on holiday

Are you off on holiday? Good for you! First of all, ignore everyone who wants to give you a horror story. This is your chance to get away and have a change of scene. Yes, there is a certain amount of stress when you travel with children, but accept that, and the rest is a bonus. Secondly, do not allow sleep stress to ruin your holiday. Even if the sleep is a mess, you're away from home, you're not working, and you're together. Decide in advance to not let your holiday be over-shadowed by bad nights or dodgy naps.

That said, I do have some practical tips to share. Mostly, concerns about travel relate to packing for little ones, travelling with small people, and time zone differences.

Packing

Personally, I'm a list girl. I like to write down what each person will need, and pack extras of the essentials. This has come from my notoriety at forgetting something important every single time I travelled with my children for the first four years. I truly mean that. Ask my husband if you don't believe me. I have forgotten underwear, nappies, shoes, coats, tooth-brushes, and pyjamas. Many of them several times over. It's cost me a fortune in unnecessary emergency shopping trips. So, having learnt the hard way, and yes, I'm a slow learner, I now write lists. Maybe you're better at this stuff than I am, or maybe you can relate – who knows. But first of all, make sure you don't forget essential things. It's so irritating! I usually pack a bag for the kids and a bag for me separately. This is because we've had the annoying experience of trying to hunt through a big communal bag in the dark, using the torch on our phones. Now, we pack our gear separately and can unpack in the light. If your baby is exclusively milk fed in a bottle, make sure you have enough milk (whether expressed or formula) to see you through your journey. Check out the rules and regulations about flying with milk on this website: www.gov.uk/hand-luggage-restrictions/baby-food-and-baby-milk. Depending on where you are travelling, you may be able to buy nappies, wipes, dummies and anything else you may have forgotten or run out of when you reach your destination. I find one of the least stressful ways to pack is to get a bag out (with my list nearby!) and start throwing things into the bag as I remember them, over a few days. But maybe you're a chuck-it-in-at-the-last-minute person. As long as you don't forget your baby, your keys, and clean underwear, there's not much that can go (seriously) wrong here.

Travelling

I vividly remember my own mother's anxiety levels rising visibly prior to travelling. As kids we never understood it – we were just excited. Now I get it. You'll either be travelling by car, boat, or plane, and usually a combination of at least two of those.

Having somehow managed to give birth to two vehement car-haters, my worst nightmare when they were little was a long car trip, but at least I have lots of tips I can share with you:

- Consider driving at bedtime or over a long nap – they may sleep through it
- Never travel hungry – recipe for disaster! But with a young baby, allow at least 30 minutes after a feed, so your baby is not curled up in their car seat with trapped gas or a dirty nappy.
- Very young children cannot tell us they feel nauseous – it is a very difficult sensation to describe. If your baby is unsettled or crying, it's certainly something to consider. Try varying when you travel, and go easy on windy roads. Pick big straight roads if you have the choice, even if it takes a little longer.
- Allow plenty of time – it *always* takes longer than you think with kids in tow.

- If your baby cries a lot in the car seat, try music (experiment with different genres), nursery rhymes, children's audio books, tell them a story out loud (make it up), children's guided meditations, or sing. I used to have to be the mummy juke box – nothing else would do.
- If your child is in a rear-facing car seat, they may like a mirror or a toy to play with to distract them.
- If you are able to, sit in the back with your little one while your partner drives.
- Plan your timing to allow for plenty of stops.

Car drives and boats are very similar, except that on a boat, you'll generally be able to walk around, which is a bonus. Flights, on the other hand, represent a whole new world of travel drama. Make sure you have the things you will need in hand luggage, and be sure to check what you can and can't take on your flight. While flying, here are some tips:

- If you're flying with a baby, you can request seats with a bassinet, to safely take off and land with your baby. It's also somewhere for them to sleep safely – in fact, they may be the only one to get a decent sleep – unless you're lucky enough to be flying business or first class.
- Your baby may want to breastfeed or suck on a dummy/pacifier during take-off and landing to ease the pressure in their ears. Older children can be allowed to suck on something else – sweets/candy are not usually the mainstay of sensible eating, but in this case they're not a bad idea.
- Bring lots of very small toys, books, and snacks.
- Bring an eye mask for yourself or your toddler to help block out the light on the aircraft.
- Bring child-size headphones – the headphones supplied on planes are usually in-ear ones, which don't work well with small children.
- Nobody will judge you if your child watches back-to-back cartoons.
- Get up and walk around the plane with your baby – it's boring and cramped for both of you.
- Take turns with your partner to settle small children on longer flights so you can each get some rest.

Travelling can be difficult – there's no doubt about it, but keep reminding yourself that it will be worth it when you arrive!

Time-zone differences

I often get asked about managing time-zone differences. My experience is actually that small time zone differences (1–2 hours), and huge ones (10–12 hours +), are the most difficult. The easiest ones seem to be the moderate time zone changes. The reason for this is that with a small time-zone change – even with daylight saving for example, the shift is so small that we sometimes just absorb it. It's no surprise that there are always hundreds of memes and posts on social media about daylight saving, because I genuinely find it to cause more problems than a more dramatic change. We forget to shift mealtimes, bedtime sneaks a little bit later, and all of a sudden you've lost that hour you were supposed to gain. Huge time-zone changes are hard because they literally flip the circadian rhythm upside down. In this scenario, it's not just a case of moving everything by five hours, or whatever, but literally reversing your entire day. That's pretty tough, and will take longer to adjust to.

My recommendation for very small time-zone differences including daylight saving, is to shift all the times in your day –meal times and wake up times. Often, things go wrong when only the bedtime is shifted. You'll need to adjust *all* your timings for this to work. You may, if it's very light, need to get creative with some tin foil or blackout blinds, or even use refuse sacks to stuff up cracks letting the light in.

The main ways to deal with a more significant time difference fall roughly into three strategies:

1. Do nothing – just stay on the home time-zone, and accept that you'll be out of sync slightly. This works best for a relatively small time-zone change, when you're planning a fairly relaxed holiday, with low expectations. It also works well if you can nap in the day to compensate for potentially early starts or late nights.
2. Make small shifts before your travel – move your entire routine by 30 minutes every couple of days, starting a few days before you travel, and then have a couple of days to continue your small shifts when you are there. This works well for very significant time-zone changes, as long as you are planning to be in your new destination for at least two weeks.
3. Just go with the flow. Stay on your home time-zone until you land, then immediately get into the new time-zone. This works best for moderate time-zone differences, and if you won't be staying very

long. You'll need to accept a dodgy day or two on arrival, and when you get home again, but this is great for people who don't want or aren't able to plan small shifts in advance.

In general, being outdoors as much as possible, eating at locally appropriate times, and being very active are your main weapons in the time-zone challenge! It is said that it takes one day to adjust per hour of time-zone change, which gives you an idea of how long it may take to really feel adjusted. Have a great holiday!

Chapter thirteen

Support yourself to better sleep

→ You may have jumped straight to this chapter. I don't blame you for that. It's natural to want to find a way out of the fatigue. While the other chapters will help you to get some clarity about your little one's sleep, I've tried to structure this chapter so that it doesn't matter if you read this first.

If you read this book in sequence, this will read like a summary, pulling together the threads of the previous chapters into a practical and implementable plan.

You may be thinking that if you are tired, and the nights are problematic, that you should work on the nights first. I put it to you that this is the hard way. It might feel logical - after all, the nights are what you need to change to get more sleep. But think about it. Doing anything other than what you're doing right now, is likely to be harder, take longer, and be less reliable. All this adds up to *even less* sleep, so it may not be something you have the capacity for right now.

Not only is changing sleep at night likely to cause more acute sleep deprivation, but being fatigued is not always directly related to your nights. That might sound equally illogical, but hear me out. Fatigue and tiredness are affected by how we feel: our confidence, our mental health and physical wellbeing.

Improving sleep by not focusing on sleep

That is why, when I support parents with sleep, I leave nights to last. The idea is that we improve absolutely everything else that we possibly can. We will chip away, making small improvements that seem unrelated to sleep initially, but I promise, by the end of a few weeks you will be feeling better, and your baby may be sleeping better as well. It's much less overwhelming this way.

The elephant in the room with sleep support is that often parents feel truly fatigued and frustrated by their sleep situation, and yet they still don't have any desire at all to make their baby upset by denying them a response. You are allowed to complain about being tired without the pressure of making changes. This is another reason for addressing aspects of your life, wellbeing and relationships before sleep. Essentially, we are hoping that sleep passively improves, spontaneously and without stress. We might not have completely resolved your sleep problem, but it is very likely that you will be feeling better, and seeing some changes and improvements.

Where to start?

I challenge you now to think about two things. Firstly, I'd like you to think about what your goals and priorities for change are. Secondly, please write down what you would like to change, and also what you definitely want to keep the same. You may want to discuss this with your co-parent, and make sure you're on the same page. Consider your compromises and your deal-breakers (See chapter eleven).

Focus on what you can control, not on what is outside your control. This might sound obvious, but I challenge you to consider the areas that you are taking responsibility for, or attempting to control, that are actually either not your responsibility, or outside your control.

For example, are you assuming responsibility for:

- How much daytime sleep your baby is getting?
- How long your baby naps?
- How long they stay asleep at night?
- Whether they even sleep at all?

I put it to you that none of these aspects of sleep are strictly within your control. However, the things that *are* in your control include:

- How you respond to your baby
- When and how you provide the conditions for sleep
- The sleep environment and location
- How you choose to feel when your child does not nap, or wakes soon after falling asleep

There will be other things that you think of. Consider carefully whether they are truly in your control or not. Remember, it is not your responsibility to make your child fall asleep, it is only your responsibility to provide the conditions, safety and responsiveness for sleep.

Next, when it is the right time for you to start to make some changes, I usually suggest you spend a few days – perhaps 3–7 days, on each of the following five distinct steps – there is some homework to do too. They may not feel relevant to sleep, but I promise, if you work through these, you will notice changes and improvements over the next few weeks:

Step 1: Understanding your child's behavioural and emotional responses

Step 2: Self-care

Step 3: Sleep hygiene

Step 4: Naps

Step 5: Bedtime

Let's get started.

Step 1: Understanding your child's behavioural and emotional responses

First, you can work on understanding your *child's cues* in a new and meaningful way. No matter how old your child is, there will be more you can notice. Paying attention to cues will have several benefits:

- Enable you to respond more accurately to your child
- Help you feel more confident
- Support the close connection you have with your child
- Allow you to discern between different needs and states
- Help you to 'catch' your child before they become dysregulated

Children have very limited abilities to regulate their emotional/behavioural states. As adults we can *self-regulate* but children gradually develop this skill, which is not thought to be completely mature until at least the age of 25 years. Until then, it is common and normal for them to need parental help in the form of *co-regulation*.

To effectively co-regulate your child, you'll need to be attuned to them – this is the ability to accurately interpret and then act on your child's emotional and behavioural clues, by moderating your behaviour, emotional state, actions and communication to meet their needs.

Different needs

You are already aware of the many ways in which your child communicates with you, whether they are verbal or not. Remember that the vast majority of our communication is non-verbal, and they will communicate many needs. Stop and consider for a few moments how your child lets you know that they are:

- Hungry
- Lonely
- Tired
- Bored
- Over-stimulated
- Scared

Your child may use a variety of communication strategies, such as speech, crying, whining, wriggling, squirming, back-arching, thumb/finger-sucking, grimacing, yawning, avoiding eye contact, losing interest in toys and surroundings and so on. I also want you to think about some specific signs your child is able to use. What does your child do to communicate the following states?

1. **When they are ready to sleep, calm and drowsy**
   Do they slow down, do they sit calmly, are they quiet and relaxed?

2. **When they are alert, playful, ready to engage or learn**
   Do they meet your eye contact, laugh, smile, concentrate on a task for a short time (this will be age-dependent)?

3. **When they are becoming upset, over-stimulated, overtired, or bored**
   Do they whine, fuss, lose interest in playing, want to be held more, raise their voice?

4. **When they are dysregulated and having a meltdown**
   Do they start to cry, shout, hit, buck/plank/arch in your arms?

Spotting behavioural and emotional states

Being able to spot what state your child is in will help you to move them from an unhelpful state into a more helpful state. Spotting what these states look like can help you understand what happened *before* they entered that state, which will help you to potentially prevent it.

Leah Kuypers refers to these states as the 'Zones of Regulation', and labels them by colour:

- When they are ready to sleep, calm and drowsy - **BLUE ZONE**
- When they are alert, playful, ready to engage or learn - **GREEN ZONE**
- When they are becoming upset, over-stimulated, overtired, or bored - **YELLOW ZONE**
- When they are dysregulated and having a meltdown - **RED ZONE**

No zone is 'bad', but understanding the emotional state can really help to understand our children's underlying needs which affect their behaviour, communication and relationships.

Triggers

If you spot that your child is in the yellow zone, what triggered them? Some possibilities are:

- Hunger
- Tiredness
- Being hot or cold
- Sensory overload – too noisy, too itchy, too tight, too dirty, too bright...
- An emotional need
- Missing someone they love
- Transitioning from one activity or environment to another
- Pain or discomfort

You might not always know what triggered your child to react the way they did, but keeping notes over a few days, observing them, noticing what keeps them **GREEN** and what makes them **YELLOW** or **RED**, will help you to understand what their behaviour is actually telling you.

Preventing red-zone behaviour

Preventing a meltdown, or even the slippery slope from yellow to red, will be your goal. This is where you get a better understanding of your child, and you are better able to meet their needs by accurately inter-preting what they are trying to tell you. Also, knowing what will send them into a dysregulated state will help you to potentially avoid these situations.

The first step is to know the triggers so you can *predict* problems. For example, do you need to adjust your child's naps? Are they waiting too long for a nap, or bedtime? Or is it too short? Is it losing focus? Has bedtime become associated with wakefulness? Can you predict what will set your child on a dysregulated path?

The next step is to have strategies for *preventing* that dysregulated behaviour. This might mean you need to change timings, locations, or avoid certain places or activities. Do you need to have a snack handy to avoid hunger meltdowns? Do you need to simplify your day? Or perhaps have a change of scene?

Helping your child

At first, you might just have to react and deal with whatever behaviour you spot. Even after you learn what triggers your child to become dysregulated, there may be times when you can't avoid a trip into the yellow zone. So you'll need to have some tricks up your sleeve to calm them down. Not all strategies will work for all children. In fact, some of the most effective strategies for one child may have the opposite effect on another. Observe your child and see which strategies are most effective for them. Remember that that the strategies that work to calm down one type of behaviour may not work in all circumstances. Keep track of what works, and you'll build up a rich picture of how to calm your child and meet their needs. Some children find the following interventions helpful:

- Firm holding, wrapping, swaddling, or wrap in a sheet or blanket with firm pressure
- Touch – stroking, massage, cuddles, head massage, hair brushing, a warm bath
- Singing, white noise, lullabies, radio, stories, absolute silence
- Take them into a dark room, take them outside in nature, lie down with them
- Sit still with them, offer them space and permission to come to you if they need to
- Food, snacks, breastfeeding, bottle-feeding, a drink

Your child

Now, I'd like you to notice what makes your child happy, sad, content, frightened, hyperactive, or distressed. Keep the following page handy and jot down anything that comes to mind over the next few days.

MY OBSERVATIONS OF MY CHILD	
BLUE ZONE **behaviour examples**	
GREEN ZONE **behaviour examples**	
YELLOW ZONE **behaviour examples**	
What happened just before? Potential triggers?	
What seems to help?	
What makes it slide into the red zone?	
RED ZONE **behaviour examples**	
What happened just before? Potential triggers?	
What seems to help?	
How did it resolve?	

Step 2: Self-care

Taking care of yourself is a really important piece of the sleep puzzle. So often, when we are tired and overwhelmed, we forget to take care of ourselves. If we can't make ourselves a priority, then you can bet your bottom dollar nobody else will. Starting today, I urge you to find ways to fill your own self-care tank.

Food and nutrition

One of the best things you can do is optimise your diet. Food isn't going to be a magic bullet, but it is true that we are what we eat. Food choices can have a big impact on our energy levels, mental fatigue and emotional well-being. Have you noticed that when you're tired you tend to eat certain foods? It's common to crave carbs and higher-fat foods which can lead to a vicious circle as these make us feel more sluggish and uncomfortable, which may worsen sleep.

I'm not saying you have to bin all the cookies, but having easily accessible healthy food is a really positive and practical thing you can do to help yourself. Stock the cupboards and fridge with healthy, feel-good food. Get easy snacks in, and plan the next week's meals. If you batch cook, try getting ahead and making some meals to save time on low-energy days.

Most of us have enough food in the freezer for at least the next two months – so you could save a fortune (and the planet) and eat up what you already have.

Finally, plan in some treats, but make this a positive choice, not something you feel guilty about. Food guilt and emotional eating is really unhelpful. If you plan for those treats you won't feel as 'naughty' for eating them.

Relationships

Our relationships with significant others can be a help or a hindrance. If your relationships prop you up and are a source of strength, compassion and support, then this is hugely helpful. If, however, the significant relationships in your life are a source of stress, then this can have a negative impact not only on your mental health, but on your sleep as well. There is solid evidence that improving the co-parenting relationship will improve both adult and child sleep. So often, becoming a parent is fraught with changes in the relationship you have with your partner. There is frequently an initial shift in the balance of power and equality in the relationship dynamic. A common response to feeling 'demoted' or 'undervalued' in the primary parenting role is to become the 'expert' on the baby. Accompanying this, according to perinatal relationship expert Elly Taylor,[1] there will often be criticising, nit-picking and exasperation as the other partner tries hard but fails to live up to the expectations of the primary caregiver. This criticism and inadvertent shaming and blaming is difficult to live with, so the other partner tends to withdraw for self-preservation. Before you know it, there is a distance in the relationship that wasn't there before.

Other relationships can suffer too – notably the relationship you have with your own parents. Becoming a parent can be very triggering for some people who don't have positive memories of being parented. Added to this, we sometimes inadvertently fall into the patterns of behaviour modelled by our parents. Just to make matters more complex, our partner will also do this – which may lead to some conflict, as you work out whose style of parenting you are trying to emulate, or how to forge your own unique way of raising your child.

Some practical pieces of advice:

- Sit down with your partner and acknowledge that the relationship has changed. Make time to listen to each other and share your feelings.
- Prioritise time together – even if it's just a quick meal with no TV distraction.
- Don't neglect touch and contact. Frequently, the primary caregiver is 'touched out' and without realising, can begin to have so many of their touch needs met (or overloaded) by their child, that they don't touch their partner. Holding hands is a good start! Or a back rub. A shoulder squeeze. You get the idea. Humans *need* touch. It's one of the ways we get a hit of oxytocin. Oxytocin isn't just important for children – adults need it to feel bonded too.
- Consciously remember to tell your partner that you value and appreciate them.
- Review your parenting goals together and make them your own.

Social support

When was the last time you chatted to a friend? Had a coffee? Went out for a meal? Are there people who you find to be a drain on your emotional energy? Do you need to duck out of social media for a while, or leave some groups? Sometimes, we need to review who we are spending most of our time with. The people you spend all your time with now may be completely different to those you spent time with before. Is this a positive change in your life? Or are you missing your old friends? Is there anything you could do about this? Scheduling a date with a friend – even if you can't make it happen for three months – will give you something to look forward to.

Emotional needs, stress and wellbeing

Our emotional health can have a big impact on our sleep, and overall well-being. Finding ways to reduce stress, manage stress and meet our needs is crucial. Children pick up on our emotional state and react to it. I don't say that to make anyone feel bad – this is normal and happens for everyone. You don't need to be on perfect form every minute of the day. But often children pick up on our anxiety, irritation and frustration with sleep. Now, let me be clear – you'd have to be superhuman not to get frustrated with sleep! But if you can be more aware of how your child's sleep makes you feel, and offload it somewhere, you'll be able to get on top of your emotional state before naps and bedtime and convey a more positive and calming state to your child. Some quick ways to calm down:

- Slow deep breaths – bringing your awareness to your breath can be really calming. Use a guided relaxation if you like – there are hundreds on YouTube.
- Try alternate nostril breathing. Close your left nostril with your finger, and exhale out of your right nostril, then inhale through the right, and then cover your right nostril while you exhale out of the left. Then inhale through your left nostril, and cover the right. Then repeat. Doing alternate nostril breathing for 5-10 minutes has been shown to reduce heart rate, blood pressure and breathing rate. So it *will* make you feel calmer. Promise.
- Try journaling – writing down how you feel, or even using a simple numeric scale to help you to feel validated, and it can be cathartic to 'dump' our thoughts on paper.
- Try listening to affirmations, guided meditations, relaxation tracks, music or nature sounds.
- Try visualisation. Imagine a calmer, more confident you, and then place that version of yourself in a scene that makes you feel calm and peaceful. Visualisation isn't for everyone, but it has been shown to be really helpful for some.

Health

Do you have unresolved issues with your health, birth story, energy levels or mental health that could be better addressed by another professional? Do you have chronic pain, inflammation, skin complaints, allergies or any other issue? I urge you to make time to deal with these issues. Pick up the phone and make that physiotherapy appointment for your bad back. Call the doctor about that thing you've been worried about for a few weeks. Take your multi-vitamins. Schedule an appointment with a psychotherapist or counsellor and make your mental health a priority. You are important – if you don't take care of yourself, your child is definitely not going to remind you to.

Exercise

Exercise releases endorphins, serotonin and keeps us fit and healthy. I know it can be really hard to find time to exercise. The logistics of finding an activity that you can do as a parent can be really off-putting. But get creative – there are plenty of things you can do that you can take your child along to. Some classes have a crèche – although this isn't for everyone, it might be an option for you. Or consider child-friendly exercise. Dance around the room with your little one, put them in a baby carrier and go for a walk, join a pushchair fit class, or go to parent and baby yoga or Pilates. It's all about finding something you *can* do. Don't stress about what you can't do.

Patience and compassion

Finally, learn to be patient. Sleep improvements take time. Give yourself permission to take the pressure off. As I have already said, you are not responsible for your child's sleep – all you have to do is provide the right conditions and environments for sleep. Having compassion for yourself, for others, and for your child will go a long way to helping your expectations to be realistic, your capacity for patience to increase, and your tolerance of your child's sleep to improve.

Step 3: Sleep hygiene

The next step is all about sleep hygiene. Sleep hygiene refers to the habits and behaviours we have before falling asleep. Good sleep hygiene means that the bedroom, bed, sleep environment, bedtime routine and even lying down are all associated with a prompt response of falling asleep. Poor sleep hygiene can cause insomnia, poor sleep quality and fragmented sleep.

How is your own sleep hygiene and why does this matter?

Whenever I work with families, I always ask them to review their own sleep hygiene first. So often we look to our children's sleeping habits as a first step. Let's face it, it is easier to change *your own* sleep than someone else's sleep, especially if that someone else is pre-verbal and lacks emotional maturity. If you can optimise your own sleep hygiene, you may find that you feel better quite quickly, without even going near your child's sleep. Even if this does not resolve your problem fully, it is likely that improving your sleep, even by a small degree, will lead to better tolerance of your child's sleep, and more energy to cope with sleep fragmentation.

* * *

SLEEP HYGIENE QUIZ

Let's start by having you take this short quiz. Tick the answer(s) that apply to you:

1. What temperature is your bedroom at night?

- 14–16°C
- 16–18°C (this is ideal)
- 18–20°C
- 20–22°C
- 22°C+

If this is a problem – what could you do about this?

2. How light is your bedroom at night?

- Pitch black (aim for total darkness if you can)
- Pretty dark
- Fairly light
- I sleep with a dim light on

If this is a problem – what action could you take?

3. Do you go to bed at roughly the same time each day?

- Yes, every day (right answer!)
- I go to bed at fairly consistent times midweek but stay up 1–2 hours later at weekends or when I have a day off the next day
- I go to bed at fairly consistent times midweek but stay up two hours or more later at weekends or when I have a day off the next day
- I go to bed at different times nearly every day

Having a consistent bedtime is really important to prevent you from feeling groggy.

4. If you have an important decision to make, how likely is it that you will lie awake thinking about it?

- Almost certain
- Likely
- Possible
- Unlikely (I try to make time to deal with intrusive thoughts *before* bed)

How could you allow space to deal with anxious thoughts? Could you keep a notebook by your bed? Could you journal? Could you use a guided relaxation before sleep?

5. Do you have a bedtime ritual?

- Yes, every night (right answer)
- Yes, most nights
- Yes, sometimes
- Hardly ever
- Never

How could yours be improved?

6. Do you take any medication that could be affecting your sleep?

- I don't take any medication
- I take herbal medication
- I take medication but there are no sleep-related side affects
- Yes, I take a medication that is known to affect sleep

It may be worth checking with your doctor to see if your medication has a side effect, or whether there is an alternative that would be less sleep-disrupting?

7. Do you exercise?

- Yes, vigorously every day (aim for this if you can – I know it's hard!)
- Yes, lightly every day
- Yes, once or twice a week
- Sometimes/I have a very active lifestyle
- Never

Being physically tired is important for sleep – how could you incorporate more exercise into your day?

8. In a typical week, do you take naps?

- Yes, every day (right answer)
- Most days
- Once or twice a week
- Hardly ever

Even lying down once per day and resting, without sleep, is restorative. Could you fit in a nap?

9. How long do you nap for?

- 30 minutes or less (this is ideal)
- 30-60 minutes
- 60 minutes or more
- I don't nap

Sleeping too long in the day can rob you of night-time sleep – just check that you're not setting yourself up for insomnia later

10. Do you do any of the following in the 2-4 hours before bed?

- Smoke
- Drink alcohol
- Drink tea or coffee
- Exercise vigorously

I'm not here to judge, but all of these can mess with your sleep. Try to shift them earlier in the day if you can.

11. Do you do any of the following in bed?
- Surf the internet
- Check your phone
- Work/study
- Watch TV
- Have long conversations with a partner

Beds are for sleep and intimacy only. Make sure your bed hasn't become a multi-functional space!

12. How long does it take you to fall asleep, or return to sleep if you are woken in the night?
- I'm asleep instantly (this suggests significant sleep deprivation)
- Probably less than 10 minutes (this indicates some sleep deprivation)
- It takes me about 15 minutes (this is ideal)
- It often takes me more than 30 minutes (this can indicate some level of anxiety)

If you fall asleep too fast, could you go to bed earlier? If you have insomnia – I have tips coming up...

* * *

What changes could you make to your own sleep hygiene?

Having done the quiz, nearly everyone finds that they could improve even one or two aspects of their own sleep. Write down the things that you could optimise here:

Action plan. To improve my own sleep hygiene I can...

- _____

- _____

- _____

What changes could you make to your child's sleep hygiene?

Now, repeat the quiz for your child. Almost all of these criteria are applicable for children too. Remember to consider where your child sleeps. If you have a nursery set up but your child is in your bedroom (as they should be if your little one is under 6-12 months) then think about *your* bedroom, not the nursery.

Action plan. To improve my child's sleep hygiene I can

- _____

- _____

- _____

Do you need to buy anything to make your life easier?

Having completed your action plan, you may find you need to make some changes. Here are some possible products that might help:

- Blackout blinds (or use aluminium foil, or black garbage sacks to stuff up any cracks. Remember that you need to do this in any room where people are sleeping)
- Lovey (this could be a muslin square, blanket or soft toy)

- Co-sleeper crib
- Baby sleeping bags
- Cotton sheets and other cool bedding
- Fan
- Dehumidifier
- White noise (try YouTube, apps or iTunes)
- Meditation tracks

In addition, you might find that you need to:

- Declutter the sleep environment
- Remove objects that might be casting scary shadows
- Switch from a blue or white light to a red nightlight which will not interfere with melatonin production

Insomnia

Finally, I promised some help with insomnia. If you find that it takes either you or your child a long time to fall asleep, then this can have a negative impact on your sleep hygiene. Taking more than 30 minutes to fall asleep could mean that the bedroom, bed, bedtime routine and sleep environment have become associated with wakefulness and alertness, and sometimes stress, arguments, procrastination or negotiation instead of a rapid onset of sleep. This can turn into a vicious circle, and instead of the sleep routine being conducive to sleep, it can trigger wakefulness and anxious thoughts. The solution is two-fold:

- Work out and address any underlying causes of stress/anxiety
- Create positive associations with the bedroom
  - No fighting
  - Gentle voices
  - Don't send children to their room as a punishment
  - Allow some happy time in the crib/cot/bed if your child has become fretful and upset when placed in their bed
- Delay bedtime until you (or your child) are genuinely very tired
  - Wait until you normally fall asleep before getting ready for bed
  - You will hopefully have a rapid onset of sleep
  - This will change the association of bed to a positive and sleepy one!

- When this has been going well for at least a week, begin going to bed earlier
- Move bedtime earlier very slowly – by 15 minutes every 2-3 days

Step 4: Naps

This step is all about naps! The purpose of a nap is to take the lid off sleep pressure, to prevent your child from becoming excessively tired. As we move through the day, we build up sleep pressure. The younger we are, the faster the sleep pressure builds. So, as an adult, you can probably tolerate being awake for anything from 14–20 hours before sleep pressure becomes extreme. Younger children build up sleep pressure much faster. Working out what your child's unique nap needs are will be the focus of this stage of the sleep coaching program. You'll need to refer back to your observations in Step 1.

Sleep gates

Sleep gates are the times when sleep pressure is high, but your little one is not yet getting cranky. Think of a pan bubbling on the stove. The sleep pressure needs to build to a point where your pan is bubbling. If there are no bubbles, your child is genuinely not tired enough for sleep. You'll get resistance and wakefulness, and this can lead to sleep and nap refusal and a negative association with the pre-sleep routine. When your child's sleep pressure is bubbling, this is the optimum time to try for a nap. You'll need to review the exercise in Step 1 when we looked at behavioural and emotional states to help you figure out how your child tells you they are tired.

Number of naps

Please take all information about nap needs with a pinch of salt. This is not designed to be taken literally, or followed exactly. As the world expert on your child, you will know if these rough guidelines apply to your child or whether your little one is an outlier. Don't be afraid to experiment. Try two naps one day, and observe to see if it seems to work, and then the next day try one nap. Every child is different. However, I am often asked for some loose suggestions, so although this can vary massively both by age, and even among children, I have found that many children find their way towards these patterns. As a rough rule, you might see:

- 0-3 months – many evenly spread naps throughout the day
- 3-6 months – often four naps
- 6-9 months – usually three naps
- 9-16 months – mostly two naps
- 16-36 months – usually one nap

Length of naps

The truth is, naps can vary in length according to your child's age, level of tiredness, and how many naps they take. The more naps your child has, the more likely they are to be short (45 minutes or less). I want to challenge you today to reframe your expectation of what 'short' means. Short naps can be great! They are restorative. Your friend's child may nap for two hours, but maybe that's what they need. It doesn't mean your child can be persuaded to do that. I'm also aware that naps are a chance to get a break from your child. I really understand that. But let's take this one step at a time.

I often suggest that you start by thinking about your child's longest potential nap. If they could choose the location of their sleep, how would they sleep? How long would they sleep? This is your child's longest possible sleep. So if your child sleeps for 90 minutes in the baby carrier, but only 20 minutes in their crib – you know that their longest potential nap is 90 minutes. If, however, they sleep for 20 minutes wherever they are, then *this* is their limit. Remember that sometimes napping too long may be the cause of night waking, or a party in the middle of the night. Try to be open-minded.

If your child wakes from a nap and you thought they would/could sleep longer, then think about the following:

- Were they in their favourite location?
- Is it possible they need fewer naps, so that they are more tired before their nap?
- How do they seem? Happy? Or cranky?
- What is the main thing that bothers you about your child's short nap?
- How do they sleep at night? Are short naps part of the problem, or does your child have short naps because they sleep well at night?
- Could you prolong the nap by hovering nearby when you think they will wake?
- Could you prolong the nap by providing the same conditions they had to fall asleep?
- Could you prolong the nap by adding in background noise?

Nap gaps

The nap gap is very personal to your child. This is the amount of time they can be awake before they get cranky. Using your work from Step 1, I'd like you to work on your child's optimal nap gaps. Remember that you'll need to be flexible – if they have a tiring day they may need a shorter nap gap. If they've had an easier day they may need a longer nap gap. If you're dropping a nap, you may need to adjust the other timings, including your bedtime.

How does my child tell me they are ready for sleep?	
How long have they been awake when they show these signs?	Shortest interval: Longest interval:
How does my child tell me they are cranky?	
How long have they been awake when they show these signs?	Shortest interval: Longest interval:
My child's approximate nap gap is:	

Location of naps

Many parents are frustrated by how or where their child sleeps for naps. Perhaps this is with motion, or perhaps they fall asleep best during a feed. I want to challenge you today to work on reframing how your child falls asleep with positive language.

Instead of: 'My child uses me as a dummy', or 'My baby only ever falls asleep when I rock them', I'd like you to think: 'I am a calm, competent, responsive parent, and I have a fool-proof way of getting my child to fall asleep'.

Now, I appreciate that the way your child falls asleep may not feel sustainable, but it is actually the first step of four. Let's review those steps to sleep:

1. You can get your child to fall asleep, in the location that works for them, and at the time that meets their needs

2. You can get your child to fall asleep, with some limits on location, at the time that works for your child

3. You can get your child to fall asleep, in the location that works for you, at the time that works for them, with lots of parental support

4. You can get your child to fall asleep, in the location that works for you, at the time that works for them, with a sustainable amount of support

When you reframe your initial mechanism for sleep as a positive, you'll see that it is a tool that you can use to move you towards your goal, rather than feeling angry or guilty about it.

Step 5: Bedtime

You are coming into land on a few weeks of hard work, making gradual, respectful and sustainable changes for you, your family and your child. We're going to dive into the nuts and bolts of bedtime now and make this as good as we can get it.

Purpose
First of all, the purpose of the bedtime routine is to create a positive, nurturing association with sleep, a loving end to the day, and an opportunity to calm down and become ready for sleep. It's also a time to connect before that long separation that comes with sleep.

I would suggest to you that you factor in some 'silly time' before your distinct wind-down for sleep. This might sound counter-intuitive, but if children have lots of pent-up energy, then you might find that bedtime doesn't go too well. Incorporating some exercise, giggling, and fun time before you start might really help you and your little one.

Timing

Many people assume that a 7pm bedtime is 'normal' or 'optimal'. When you work out a bedtime for your child, you'll need to consider:

- What is culturally normal for you – in many cultures, a later bedtime is normal
- When your child has to get up the next day – do they have enough opportunity to get enough sleep for them? Remember that for many children, 10-11 hours of sleep at night is pretty normal. So, factor this in when you're thinking about a suitable bedtime. If your child usually wakes up at 6am, then realistically, a bedtime of 8pm may be appropriate. A bedtime that is too early may lead to a very early start.
- What time are your naps – are they spaced in such a way that fits with bedtime? Are there large gaps that allow your child to become overtired or cranky?
- What suits your family, lifestyle, working patterns and family mealtimes?

An 'earlier bedtime' is not intended to mean a particular time, it simply means 'earlier than right now'.

Sequence and content

Doing the same things in the same order enables your child to learn to predict what will happen next. Don't be afraid to listen to your child and find out what makes them calm. Review your work from Step 1 and notice what makes your child upset or stressed. If a bath makes your child scream when they exit the water, then maybe abandon the bath. If certain stories make your child too excited, then forget them and choose an alternative.

Here are some popular activities to include – but remember that the activities that one child finds soothing may cause another child stress or too much excitement:

- Bath
- Stories
- Cuddle
- Feed
- Snack
- Massage
- Song
- Quiet play
- Meditation tracks
- Prayer

What activities make my child excited or stressed?

- _____
- _____
- _____

Activities my child finds soothing	How long does this activity take?

When you work out which activities your child likes and doesn't like, you'll narrow down what to include in your bedtime routine. Then, you'll probably need to narrow it down further to make it a suitable length. For example, if your child likes a bath (20 minutes) massage (20 minutes) stories (10 minutes) and feed (30 minutes) then your bedtime routine may get too long. You may need to either shorten an activity or do it at another time.

Length

The length of your bedtime routine will depend on your child's age and attention span. Don't be afraid to adjust the length according to their need. If they don't seem to be tired, you can delay it, or extend it. If they are very tired, start bedtime early, or make it shorter, either by skipping a step, or condensing the steps. A good maximum length is about 45 minutes after about 6-9 months of age. Younger babies will probably need a much shorter routine than this.

People involved

Often, a child will come to expect or prefer one parent over another. This can be really demoralising for both parents. One parent feels overwhelmed and potentially touched out, and the other feels rejected. One option, rather than 'forcing' a child to have the 'other' parent, is to have both parents do bedtime. Lots of parents find that having the 'other' parent passive but present is a good first step. Then the passive parent can become progressively more involved as the days go by and as the child begins to adjust and associate the other parent with bedtime. Then, ultimately, the more active parent becomes more passive.

Location

Where the bedtime routine happens can be really important. Starting in the bedroom and migrating to the living area can cause your child to become excited again. Try to stay in the 'quiet' zone once bedtime has begun.

However, you might want to consider giving your bedtime routine a head start by dimming the lights, quietening voices, changing the type of activity and reducing exposure to screens and stimulation in the living area before you start bedtime. This gives your child an opportunity to start to calm down before bedtime.

Attitude

Being positive, nurturing, and emotionally available is really important. I often say that bedtime can feel like the 'gutter' of the day. Everyone is tired, and as parents we are often ready to be finished with parenting after a long day. Acknowledge that and allow yourself to feel this if this applies to you. That's okay. It doesn't make you a bad parent! But if you can acknowledge it, dump it somewhere, and then dig deep and find your last scraps of energy from somewhere, you'll find that being gentle, patient and responsive at bedtime will help bedtime to be more peaceful and efficient. Review your tools from Step 2 and use those here as well.

We can also take time to understand that for our children, bedtime is a time of separation and loss. Connecting with them, and filling their love tank before this separation, will help to stop them from seeking more of us in the night to compensate for missing us in the day.

Realistic expectations

Finally, making time to check our expectations can reduce disappointment and frustration. Think about having a realistic time frame for improvements. This is strongly related to habits – which can take several weeks to be established. Change is hard, which is why adding a new and more sustainable habit cannot often instantly replace an existing habit. But one thing that you could do is to try a strategy such as 'habit stacking'. This is where you add a new habit to an existing and well-established one. For example, if your child feeds to sleep, if you replace this with patting, it is likely to end in tears. But if you add patting *on top of* feeding to sleep, your child may come to associate those two behaviours with falling asleep. It takes time to stack new habits, but this can be a very effective and gentle strategy.

What next?

After a few weeks of gently addressing sleep around the outside, it's a good idea to take stock. What is better? What hasn't changed? Do you feel like you are now in a place where you can just let your child's sleep evolve? Or is your sleep situation still unmanageable? You can go back to the strategies in chapter ten and eleven and see if one of those might be a good fit for your family.

I wish you lots of luck!

Conclusion

→ As a new parent, it's likely that you have heard many different ideas and theories about sleep. It often feels like the definition of parental success is having a 'good baby'. A 'good baby' is a 'good sleeper' – one who wakes infrequently and needs little intervention.

The truth is, that not only is sleep not the measure of your parenting, but it is also not necessarily something that you as a parent are wholly in control of. This idea does both parents and babies a great disservice. Babies are more than the measure of how they live up to objective and measurable criteria, and parents are worth so much more than their apparent 'success' in achieving a certain number of hours of sleep. If this was the main feature of successful parenting, then the hard work would be largely over before a child goes to preschool. Don't let anyone minimise your role to 'sleep achiever'. You are worth far more than that.

It can also feel like the key to this desirable good sleeper is a closely guarded secret. I assure you that if there was an easy, quick, reliable and cry-free way of helping all children sleep in a particular way, or through the night, it would be easily google-able, or you would have heard about it. I certainly do not make any sleep strategy a secret, and I do not reserve the most effective sleep tools only for my private clients.

Honestly, if you do nothing, your child will eventually sleep. If you bed-share, breastsleep, cuddle, nurture and respond your way through the first year or two (or more), your child will one day, without you doing anything clever or difficult, just drift off to sleep. If you want or need to make sleep more sustainable, that is totally your choice, but please do not feel that this is somehow a kind of rite of passage or an inevitable feature of parenting.

If you take nothing else away from this book, my sincere hope is that you feel you have a better, more complete, and realistic picture of sleep, and the role that responsive parenting has to play within this. I also hope you know that you are not alone, your child is not broken, and you are not failing.

Whether you make a positive and informed choice to do nothing, instigate some gentle and sustainable strategies to make sleep more bearable, or choose to embark on changing the way bedtime works, I wish you every success not just in sleep, but mostly in your journey as a parent.

Acknowledgements

I have wanted to write a book for parents about sleep for years. I hesitated because many people have published a sleep 'method', a mnemonic to remember the steps, or a diagram to succinctly outline the strategies. I have no methods, or mnemonics. No diagrams either for that matter. I worried that people wouldn't understand that I am trying to walk in a murky, difficult place where I hold multiple realities as truth simultaneously. The reality that I firmly uphold gentle, responsive parenting. The reality of biologically normal aspects of infant sleep and development. The reality of the overwhelm, exhaustion and confusion of parents, and the multiple voices claiming to know the secrets of sleeping babies. These cannot be distilled into a 3-step plan. At the simplest level, what I promote is not one single method, but a practical interpretation of the tools which may work, based on the best available evidence at the time, sifted from the myriad options to include only those which are respectful, responsive and kind to babies and families. It's not easy to wade in this area, but for me, it's worth it.

For the hundreds of professionals and parents who asked me to write this book, this is for you. I have tried to download my brain - I hope this was what you wanted and needed. Sorry it took me so long.

To my two girls, both of whom have taught me the brutal reality of exhaustion, but showed me that all annoying phases do indeed come to an end, thank you for the fabulous people you are turning out to be. Thanks to my parents for being 1980s rebels and raising me responsively - you're legends.

Finally, thank you to the team at Pinter & Martin for seeing my vision. Here's to the next one!

References

Chapter 1: Addressing sleep myths

1. Howson, S. (2018). 'I See No Other Option.' Maternal Practices of Sleep-Training and Co-Sleeping as the Management of Vulnerability. *Studies in the Maternal, 10*(1).

2. Brown, A., & Harries, V. (2015). Infant sleep and night feeding patterns during later infancy: Association with breastfeeding frequency, daytime complementary food intake, and infant weight. *Breastfeeding Medicine, 10*(5), 246-252.

3. Dupont, D., Ménard, O., & Deglaire, A. (2018, November). Differences in composition and structure between human milk and infant formula: do they affect their digestion?. In *15. International Symposium on Milk Genomics and Human Health* (p. np).

4. Gridneva, Z., Kuganananthan, S., Hepworth, A., Tie, W., Lai, C., Ward, L., ... & Geddes, D. (2017). Effect of human milk appetite hormones, macronutrients, and infant characteristics on gastric emptying and breastfeeding patterns of term fully breastfed infants. *Nutrients, 9*(1), 15.

5. Kent, J.C., Mitoulas, L.R., Cregan, M.D., Ramsay, D.T., Doherty, D.A. and Hartmann, P.E., (2006). Volume and frequency of breastfeedings and fat content of breast milk throughout the day. *Pediatrics, 117*(3), pp.e387-e395.

6. Hörnell, A., Aarts, C., Kylberg, E., Hofvander, Y. and Gebre-Medhin, M., (1999). Breastfeeding patterns in exclusively breastfed infants: a longitudinal prospective study in Uppsala, Sweden. *Acta paediatrica, 88*(2), pp.203-211.

7. Gridneva, Z., Kuganananthan, S., Hepworth, A., Tie, W., Lai, C., Ward, L., ... & Geddes, D. (2017). Effect of human milk appetite hormones, macronutrients, and infant characteristics on gastric emptying and breastfeeding patterns of term fully breastfed infants. *Nutrients, 9*(1), 15.

8. Canapari, C. (2019). *It's Never Too Late To Sleep Train.*

9. Cong, Z., Hale, T., & Kendall-Tackett, K. (2011). The Effect of Feeding Method on Sleep Duration, Maternal Well. being, and Pospartum Depression. *Clinical Lactation, 2*(2), 22-26.

10. Gridneva, Z., Kuganananthan, S., Hepworth, A., Tie, W., Lai, C., Ward, L., ... & Geddes, D. (2017). Effect of human milk appetite hormones, macronutrients, and infant characteristics on gastric emptying and breastfeeding patterns of term fully breastfed infants. *Nutrients, 9*(1), 15.

11. Perkin, M. R., Bahnson, H. T., Logan, K., Marrs, T., Radulovic, S., Craven, J., ... & Lack, G. (2018). Association of early introduction of solids with infant sleep: a secondary analysis of a randomized clinical trial. *JAMA pediatrics, 172*(8), e180739-e180739.

12. Brown, A., & Harries, V. (2015). Infant sleep and night feeding patterns during later infancy: Association with breastfeeding frequency, daytime complementary food intake, and infant weight. *Breastfeeding Medicine, 10*(5), 246-252.

13. Ball, H.L., (2003). Breastfeeding, bed-sharing, and infant sleep. *Birth, 30*(3), pp.181-188.

14. Butte, N.F., Jensen, C.L., Moon, J.K., Glaze, D.G. and Frost, J.D., (1992). Sleep

organization and energy expenditure of breast-fed and formula-fed infants. *Pediatric research, 32*(5), pp.514-519.

15. Brown, A., & Harries, V. (2015). Infant sleep and night feeding patterns during later infancy: Association with breastfeeding frequency, daytime complementary food intake, and infant weight. *Breastfeeding Medicine, 10*(5), 246-252.

16. Rudzik, A.E., Robinson-Smith, L., & Ball, H. L. (2018). Discrepancies in maternal reports of infant sleep vs. actigraphy by mode of feeding. *Sleep medicine, 49*, 90-98.

17. Kendall-Tackett, K., Cong, Z. and Hale, T.W., (2011). The effect of feeding method on sleep duration, maternal well-being, and postpartum depression. *Clinical Lactation, 2*(2), pp.22-26.

18. Bowlby, J. (1955). (b) The Growth of Independence in the Young Child. *Journal (Royal Society of Health), 76*(9), 587-591.

19. Mao, A., Burnham, M.M., Goodlin-Jones, B.L., Gaylor, E.E., Anders, T.F. A comparison of the sleep-wake patterns of cosleeping and solitarysleeping infants. *Child Psychiatry Hum Dev* 2004;35:95e105.

20. Mileva-Seitz, V. R., Bakermans-Kranenburg, M. J., Battaini, C., & Luijk, M. P. (2017). Parent-child bed-sharing: the good, the bad, and the burden of evidence. *Sleep Medicine Reviews, 32*, 4-27.

21. Kendall-Tackett, K., Cong, Z. and Hale, T.W., (2011). The effect of feeding method on sleep duration, maternal well-being, and postpartum depression. *Clinical Lactation, 2*(2), pp.22-26.

22. Holt, L. (1855) *The Care and Feeding of Children.* D Appleton and Company. New York and London.

23. Tomori, C. (2017). Changing cultures of nighttime breastfeeding and sleep in the US. In Dowling S., Pontin D., & Boyer K. (Eds.), *Social experiences of breastfeeding: Building bridges between research, policy and practice.*

24. Stearns, P.N., Rowland, P., & Giarnella, L. (1996). Children's sleep: Sketching historical change. *Journal of Social History*, 345-366.

25. Maute, M., & Perren, S. (2018). Ignoring Children's Bedtime Crying: The Power Of Western-Oriented Beliefs. *Infant mental health journal, 39*(2), 220-230.

26. Watson, J.B. (1913). Psychology as the behaviorist views it. *Psychological Review*, 20, 158-177.

27. Blunden, S.L., Thompson, K.R., & Dawson, D. (2011). Behavioural sleep treatments and night time crying in infants: challenging the status quo. *Sleep medicine reviews, 15*(5), 327-334.

28. Whittingham, K., & Douglas, P. (2014). Optimizing parent-infant sleep from birth to 6 months: A new paradigm. *Infant mental health journal, 35*(6), 614-623.

29. Smithson, L., Baird, T., Tamana, S., Lau, A., Mariasine, J., Chikuma, J., ... & Sears, M. R. (2018). Shorter sleep duration is associated with reduced cognitive development at 2 years of age. *Sleep medicine.*

30. Scher, A. (2005). Infant sleep at 10 months of age as a window to cognitive development. *Early Human Development, 81*(3), 289-292.

31. Gibson, R., Elder, D., & Gander, P. (2012). Actigraphic sleep and developmental progress of one-year-old infants. *Sleep and Biological Rhythms, 10*(2), 77-83.

32. Tham, E., Broekman, B., Goh, D., Teoh, O., Chong, Y., Gluckman, P., ... & Gooley, J.

(2015). Nocturnal wakefulness at 3 months predicts toddler cognitive, language and motor abilities. *Sleep Medicine, 16*, S48.

33. Pennestri, M.H., Laganière, C., Bouvette-Turcot, A.A., Pokhvisneva, I., Steiner, M., Meaney, M.J., ... & Mavan Research Team. (2018). Uninterrupted Infant Sleep, Development, and Maternal Mood. *Pediatrics*, e20174330.

34. Mindell, J.A., Leichman, E.S., DuMond, C., & Sadeh, A. (2017). Sleep and social-emotional development in infants and toddlers. *Journal of Clinical Child & Adolescent Psychology, 46*(2), 236-246.

35. Mindell, J.A., & Lee, C. (2015). Sleep, mood, and development in infants. *Infant behavior and development, 41*, 102-107.

36. Sun, W., Li, S. X., Jiang, Y., Xu, X., Spruyt, K., Zhu, Q., ... & Jiang, F. (2018). A Community-Based Study of Sleep and Cognitive Development in Infants and Toddlers. *Journal of Clinical Sleep Medicine, 14*(06), 977-984.

Chapter 2: The truth about sleep

1. Harries, V., & Brown, A. (2017). The association between use of infant parenting books that promote strict routines, and maternal depression, self-efficacy, and parenting confidence. *Early Child Development and Care*, 1-12.

2. Thomas, A., Chess, S., Birch, H. G., Hertzig, M. E., & Korn, S. (1963). Behavioral individuality in early childhood.

3. Hookway, L. (2019). Holistic Sleep Coaching. Gentle Alternatives to Sleep Training for Health and Childcare Professionals. Praeclarus Press: Amarillo

4. Ansfield, M.E., Wegner, D.M., & Bowser, R. (1996). Ironic effects of sleep urgency. *Behaviour Research and Therapy, 34*(7), 523-531.

5. Hanlon, E., Vyazovskiy, V., Faraguna, U., Tononi, G., & Cirelli, C. (2011). Synaptic potentiation and sleep need: clues from molecular and electrophysiological studies. *Current topics in medicinal chemistry, 11*(19), 2472-2482.

6. Anders, T.F. (1979). Night-waking in infants during the first year of life. *Pediatrics, 63*(6), 860-864.

7. Rothbart, M.K., Ziaie, H., & O'boyle, C.G. (1992). Self-regulation and emotion in infancy. *New directions for child and adolescent development, 1992*(55), 7-23.

8. Rothbart, M.K., Ellis, L.K., & Posner, M.I. (2004). Temperament and self-regulation. *Handbook of self-regulation: Research, theory, and applications, 2*, 441-460.

9. Owens, J.A. (2004). Sleep in children: Cross-cultural perspectives. *Sleep and Biological Rhythms, 2*(3), 165-173.

10. Leger, D., Poursain, B., Neubauer, D., & Uchiyama, M. (2008). An international survey of sleeping problems in the general population. *Current medical research and opinion, 24*(1), 307-317.

11. Mindell, J.A., Sadeh, A., Wiegand, B., How, T.H., & Goh, D.Y. (2010). Cross-cultural differences in infant and toddler sleep. *Sleep medicine, 11*(3), 274-280.

12. Sadeh, A., Mindell, J., & Rivera, L. (2011). 'My child has a sleep problem': a cross-cultural comparison of parental definitions. *Sleep medicine, 12*(5), 478-482.

13. Teti, D.M., Kim, B.R., Mayer, G., Countermine, M. Maternal emotional availability at bedtime predicts infant sleep quality. *Journal of Family Psychology*.

(2010);24:307-315.

14. Philbrook, L.E., & Teti, D.M. (2016). Bidirectional associations between bedtime parenting and infant sleep: Parenting quality, parenting practices, and their interaction. *Journal of Family Psychology*, *30*(4), 431.

15. Pennestri, M.H., Laganière, C., Bouvette-Turcot, A.A., Pokhvisneva, I., Steiner, M., Meaney, M.J., ... & Mavan Research Team. (2018). Uninterrupted Infant Sleep, Development, and Maternal Mood. *Pediatrics*, e20174330.

16. Mindell, J.A., Leichman, E.S., DuMond, C., & Sadeh, A. (2017). Sleep and social-emotional development in infants and toddlers. *Journal of Clinical Child & Adolescent Psychology*, *46*(2), 236-246.

17. Mindell, J A., & Lee, C. (2015). Sleep, mood, and development in infants. *Infant behavior and development*, *41*, 102-107.

18. Sun, W., Li, S.X., Jiang, Y., Xu, X., Spruyt, K., Zhu, Q., ... & Jiang, F. (2018). A Community-Based Study of Sleep and Cognitive Development in Infants and Toddlers. *Journal of Clinical Sleep Medicine*, *14*(06), 977-984.

19. Henderson, J.M.T., France, K.G., Owens, J.L., Blampied, N.M. Sleeping through the night: The development of self-regulated nocturnal sleep during infancy. Pediatrics. (2010);126:e1081-1087

20. Galland, B.C., Taylor, B.J., Elder, D.E., Herbison, P. Normal sleep patterns in infants and children: A systematic review of observational studies. *Sleep Medicine Reviews*. (2012);16:213-222.

21. Grille, R. (2008). *Parenting for a Peaceful World*.

22. Armstrong, M.I., Birnie-Lefcovitch, S., & Ungar, M.T. (2005). Pathways between social support, family wellbeing, quality of parenting, and child resilience: What we know. *Journal of child and family studies*, *14*(2), 269-281.

23. Leahy-Warren, P., McCarthy, G., & Corcoran, P. (2012). First-time mothers: social support, maternal parental self-efficacy and postnatal depression. *Journal of clinical nursing*, *21*(3-4), 388-397.

24. Suzuki, S. (2010). The effects of marital support, social network support, and parenting stress on parenting: Self-efficacy among mothers of young children in Japan. *Journal of Early Childhood Research*, *8*(1), 40-66.

25. Gao, L.L., Sun, K., & Chan, S.W.C. (2014). Social support and parenting self-efficacy among Chinese women in the perinatal period. *Midwifery*, *30*(5), 532-538.

Chapter 3: Optimising parent sleep

1. Dauvilliers, Y., & Tafti, M. (2008). The genetic basis of sleep disorders. *Current pharmaceutical design*, *14*(32), 3386-3395.

2. Gehrman, P.R., Keenan, B.T., Byrne, E.M., & Pack, A.I. (2015). Genetics of sleep disorders. *Psychiatric Clinics*, *38*(4), 667-681.

3. Kalmbach, D.A., Schneider, L.D., Cheung, J., Bertrand, S.J., Kariharan, T., Pack, A.I., & Gehrman, P.R. (2017). Genetic basis of chronotype in humans: Insights from three landmark GWAS. *Sleep*, *40*(2).

4. Jagannath, A., Taylor, L., Wakaf, Z., Vasudevan, S.R., & Foster, R.G. (2017). The

genetics of circadian rhythms, sleep and health. *Human molecular genetics*, *26*(R2), R128-R138.

5. Morales-Lara, D., De-la-Peña, C., & Murillo-Rodríguez, E. (2018). Dad's snoring may have left molecular scars in your DNA: the emerging role of epigenetics in sleep disorders. *Molecular neurobiology*, *55*(4), 2713-2724.

6. Narwade, S.C., Mallick, B.N., & Deobagkar, D.D. (2017). Transcriptome analysis reveals altered expression of memory and neurotransmission associated genes in the REM sleep deprived rat brain. *Frontiers in molecular neuroscience*, *10*, 67.

7. Wang, J., Pasinetti, G.M., et al. (2018). Epigenetic modulation of inflammation and synaptic plasticity promotes resilience against stress in mice. *Nature Communications*, *9*(1). DOI: 10.1038/s41467-017-02794-5.

8. Huang, H., Zhu, Y., Eliot, M.N., Knopik, V.S., McGeary, J.E., Carskadon, M.A., & Hart, A.C. (2017). Combining human epigenetics and sleep studies in Caenorhabditis elegans: a cross-species approach for finding conserved genes regulating sleep. *Journal of Sleep and Sleep Disorders Research*, *40*(6), zsx063.

9. Qureshi, I.A., & Mehler, M.F. (2014). Epigenetics of sleep and chronobiology. *Current neurology and neuroscience reports*, *14*(3), 432.

10. Breus, M. (2016). *The Power of When: Discover Your Chronotype and Maximise Your Potential*. Random House.

11. Owens, J.A., Dearth-Wesley, T., Lewin, D., Gioia, G., & Whitaker, R.C. (2016). Self-regulation and sleep duration, sleepiness, and chronotype in adolescents. *Pediatrics*, *138*(6), e20161406.

12. Jones, S.E., Lane, J.M., Wood, A.R., Van Hees, V.T., Tyrrell, J., Beaumont, R.N., ... & Tuke, M.A. (2019). Genome-wide association analyses of chronotype in 697,828 individuals provides insights into circadian rhythms. *Nature communications*, *10*(1), 343.

13. Roenneberg, T., & Merrow, M. (2016). The circadian clock and human health. *Current biology*, *26*(10), R432-R443.

14. Kendall-Tackett, K.A. (2016). *Depression in new mothers: Causes, consequences and treatment alternatives*. Routledge.

15. Kendall-Tackett, K., Cong, Z., & Hale, T. (2018). The Impact of Feeding Method and Infant Sleep Location on Mother/Infant Sleep, Maternal Depression, and Mothers' Well-Being. *Clinical Lactation*, *9*(3), 117-124.

16. Lawson, A., Murphy, K.E., Sloan, E., Uleryk, E., Dalfen, A., (2015) The relationship between sleep and postpartum mental disorders: A systematic review. *Journal of Affective Disorders*, 176:65-77.

17. Bais, B., Lindeboom, R., van Ravesteyn, L., Tulen, J., Hoogendijk, W., Lambregtse-van den Berg, M., & Kamperman, A. (2019). The Impact of Objective and Subjective Sleep Parameters on Depressive Symptoms during Pregnancy in Women with a Mental Disorder: An Explorative Study. *International journal of environmental research and public health*, *16*(9), 1587.

18. Kalmbach, D.A., Anderson, J.R., & Drake, C.L. (2018). The impact of stress on sleep: Pathogenic sleep reactivity as a vulnerability to insomnia and circadian disorders. *Journal of Sleep Research*, *27*(6), e12710.

19. Hookway, L. (2019). Holistic Sleep Coaching. Gentle Alternatives to Sleep Training

for Health and Childcare Professionals. Praeclarus Press: Amarillo

20. Butler, E.A., & Randall, A.K. (2013). Emotional coregulation in close relationships. *Emotion Review*, 5(2), 202-210.

21. Gordon, A.M., & Chen, S. (2014). The role of sleep in interpersonal conflict: do sleepless nights mean worse fights?. *Social Psychological and Personality Science*, 5(2), 168-175.

22. Morgan, M. (2018). How couple therapists work with parenting issues. In *How Couple Relationships Shape Our World* (pp. 71-84). Routledge.

23. Yarwood, G.A., & Locke, A. (2016). Work, parenting and gender: the care–work negotiations of three couple relationships in the UK. *Community, Work & Family*, 19(3), 362-377.

24. Bonvanie, I.J., Oldehinkel, A.J., Rosmalen, J.G., & Janssens, K.A. (2016). Sleep problems and pain: a longitudinal cohort study in emerging adults. *Pain*, 157(4), 957-963.

25. Dolezal, B.A., Neufeld, E.V., Boland, D.M., Martin, J.L., & Cooper, C.B. (2017). Interrelationship between sleep and exercise: a systematic review. *Advances in preventive medicine*, 2017.

26. Katagiri, R., Asakura, K., Kobayashi, S., Suga, H., & Sasaki, S. (2014). Low intake of vegetables, high intake of confectionery, and unhealthy eating habits are associated with poor sleep quality among middle-aged female Japanese workers. *Journal of occupational health*, 14-0051.

27. Schneider, N., Mutungi, G., & Cubero, J. (2018). Diet and nutrients in the modulation of infant sleep: A review of the literature. *Nutritional neuroscience*, 21(3), 151-161.

28. Lillehei, A.S., & Halcon, L.L. (2014). A systematic review of the effect of inhaled essential oils on sleep. *The Journal of Alternative and Complementary Medicine*, 20(6), 441-451.

29. Hwang, E., & Shin, S. (2015). The effects of aromatherapy on sleep improvement: a systematic literature review and meta-analysis. *The Journal of Alternative and Complementary Medicine*, 21(2), 61-68.

30. Irish, L.A., Kline, C.E., Gunn, H.E., Buysse, D.J., & Hall, M.H. (2015). The role of sleep hygiene in promoting public health: A review of empirical evidence. *Sleep medicine reviews*, 22, 23-36.

31. Taylor, D.J., Lichstein, K.L., Durrence, H.H., Reidel, B.W., & Bush, A.J. (2005). Epidemiology of insomnia, depression, and anxiety. *Sleep*, 28(11), 1457-1464.

32. Gallaher, K.G.H., Slyepchenko, A., Frey, B.N., Urstad, K., & Dørheim, S.K. (2018). The Role of Circadian Rhythms in Postpartum Sleep and Mood. *Sleep medicine clinics*, 13(3), 359-374.

33. van Straten, A., van der Zweerde, T., Kleiboer, A., Cuijpers, P., Morin, C.M., & Lancee, J. (2018). Cognitive and behavioral therapies in the treatment of insomnia: A meta-analysis. *Sleep Medicine Reviews*, 38, 3-16.

34. Saletin, J.M., Hilditch, C.J., Dement, W.C., & Carskadon, M.A. (2017). Short daytime naps briefly attenuate objectively measured sleepiness under chronic sleep restriction. *Sleep*, 40(9).

35. Tietzel, A.J., & Lack, L.C. (2001). The short-term benefits of brief and long naps following nocturnal sleep restriction. *Sleep*, 24(3), 293-300.

36. Milner, C.E., & Cote, K.A. (2009). Benefits of napping in healthy adults: impact of nap length, time of day, age, and experience with napping. *Journal of sleep research, 18*(2), 272-281.

Chapter 4: Positive sleep starts in pregnancy

1. Napso, T., Yong, H.E., Lopez-Tello, J., & Sferruzzi-Perri, A.N. (2018). The role of placental hormones in mediating maternal adaptations to support pregnancy and lactation. *Frontiers in physiology, 9.*

2. Giallo, R., Seymour, M., Dunning, M., Cooklin, A., Loutzenhiser, L., & McAuslan, P. (2015). Factors associated with the course of maternal fatigue across the early postpartum period. *Journal of reproductive and infant psychology, 33*(5), 528-544.

3. Catalano, P.M. (1999). Pregnancy and lactation in relation to range of acceptable carbohydrate and fat intake. *European Journal of Clinical Nutrition, 53*(s1), s124.

4. Taousani, E., Savvaki, D., Tsirou, E., Poulakos, P., Mintziori, G., Zafrakas, M., ... & Goulis, D. G. (2017). Regulation of basal metabolic rate in uncomplicated pregnancy and in gestational diabetes mellitus. *Hormones, 16*(3), 235-250.

5. Rukuni, R., Knight, M., Murphy, M.F., Roberts, D., & Stanworth, S.J. (2015). Screening for iron deficiency and iron deficiency anaemia in pregnancy: a structured review and gap analysis against UK national screening criteria. *BMC pregnancy and childbirth, 15*(1), 269.

6. Bai, G., Raat, H., Jaddoe, V.W., Mautner, E., & Korfage, I.J. (2018). Trajectories and predictors of women's health-related quality of life during pregnancy: A large longitudinal cohort study. *PloS one, 13*(4), e0194999.

7. Munoz-Suano, A., Hamilton, A.B., & Betz, A.G. (2011). Gimme shelter: the immune system during pregnancy. *Immunological reviews, 241*(1), 20-38.

8. Mor, G., & Cardenas, I. (2010). The immune system in pregnancy: a unique complexity. *American journal of reproductive immunology, 63*(6), 425-433.

9. Milrad, S.F., Hall, D.L., Jutagir, D.R., Lattie, E.G., Ironson, G.H., Wohlgemuth, W., ... & Fletcher, M.A. (2017). Poor sleep quality is associated with greater circulating pro-inflammatory cytokines and severity and frequency of chronic fatigue syndrome/myalgic encephalomyelitis (CFS/ME) symptoms in women. *Journal of neuroimmunology, 303*, 43-50.

10. Kendall-Tackett, K. (2015). The new paradigm for depression in new mothers: current findings on maternal depression, breastfeeding and resiliency across the lifespan. *Breastfeeding Review, 23*(1), 7.

11. Groer, M.E., Jevitt, C., & Ji, M. (2015). Immune changes and dysphoric moods across the postpartum. *American Journal of Reproductive Immunology, 73*(3), 193-198.

12. Inanir, S., Cakmak, B., Nacar, M. C., Guler, A.E., & Inanir, A. (2015). Body Image perception and self-esteem during pregnancy. *International Journal of Women's health and Reproductive Sciences,* 3 (4), 196-200

13. Neiterman, E., & Fox, B. (2017). Controlling the unruly maternal body: Losing and gaining control over the body during pregnancy and the postpartum period. *Social Science & Medicine, 174*, 142-148.

14. Brown, A., Rance, J., & Warren, L. (2015). Body image concerns during pregnancy are associated with a shorter breast feeding duration. *Midwifery, 31*(1), 80-89.

15. Roomruangwong, C., Kanchanatawan, B., Sirivichayakul, S., & Maes, M. (2017). High incidence of body image dissatisfaction in pregnancy and the postnatal period: Associations with depression, anxiety, body mass index and weight gain during pregnancy. *Sexual & Reproductive Healthcare, 13*, 103-109.

16. O'Leary, K., Dockray, S., & Hammond, S. (2016). Positive prenatal well-being: conceptualising and measuring mindfulness and gratitude in pregnancy. *Archives of women's mental health, 19*(4), 665-673.

17. Yalda Afshar MD, PHD, Nguyen, M.L., Mei, J., & Grisales, T. (2017). Sexual health and function in pregnancy. *Contemporary Ob/Gyn, 62*(8), 24.

18. Yıldız, H. (2015). The relation between prepregnancy sexuality and sexual function during pregnancy and the postpartum period: a prospective study. *Journal of sex & marital therapy, 41*(1), 49-59.

19. Polomeno, V., Bouchard, L., & Reissing, E. (2016). What do we know about perinatal sexuality? A scoping review on sexoperinatality-Part 1. *Journal de gynecologie, obstetrique et biologie de la reproduction, 45*(8), 796-808.

20. Bai, G., Korfage, I.J., Hafkamp-de Groen, E., Jaddoe, V.W., Mautner, E., & Raat, H. (2016). Associations between nausea, vomiting, fatigue and health-related quality of life of women in early pregnancy: the generation R study. *PloS one, 11*(11), e0166133.

21. Staneva, A.A., Bogossian, F., & Wittkowski, A. (2015). The experience of psychological distress, depression, and anxiety during pregnancy: A meta-synthesis of qualitative research. *Midwifery, 31*(6), 563-573.

22. Deklava, L., Lubina, K., Circenis, K., Sudraba, V., & Millere, I. (2015). Causes of anxiety during pregnancy. *Procedia-Social and Behavioral Sciences, 205*, 623-626.

23. Brunton, R.J., Dryer, R., Saliba, A., & Kohlhoff, J. (2015). Pregnancy anxiety: A systematic review of current scales. *Journal of affective disorders, 176*, 24-34.

24. Bai, G., Korfage, I.J., Hafkamp-de Groen, E., Jaddoe, V.W., Mautner, E., & Raat, H. (2016). Associations between nausea, vomiting, fatigue and health-related quality of life of women in early pregnancy: the generation R study. *PloS one, 11*(11), e0166133.

25. McParlin, C., O'Donnell, A., Robson, S.C., Beyer, F., Moloney, E., Bryant, A., ... & Norman, J. (2016). Treatments for hyperemesis gravidarum and nausea and vomiting in pregnancy: a systematic review. *Jama, 316*(13), 1392-1401.

26. Heitmann, K., Svendsen, H.C., Sporsheim, I.H., & Holst, L. (2016). Nausea in pregnancy: attitudes among pregnant women and general practitioners on treatment and pregnancy care. *Scandinavian journal of primary health care, 34*(1), 13-20.

27. Fateme, B., Fatemeh, M.K., Vahid, M., Arezou, N.J., Manizhe, N., & Zahra, M. (2019). The effect of Benson's muscle relaxation technique on severity of pregnancy nausea. *Electronic Journal of General Medicine, 16*(2).

28. McParlin, C., O'Donnell, A., Robson, S.C., Beyer, F., Moloney, E., Bryant, A., ... & Norman, J. (2016). Treatments for hyperemesis gravidarum and nausea and vomiting in pregnancy: a systematic review. *Jama, 316*(13), 1392-1401.

29. Mindell, J.A., Cook, R.A., & Nikolovski, J. (2015). Sleep patterns and sleep disturbances across pregnancy. *Sleep medicine, 16*(4), 483-488.

30. Genesoni, L., & Tallandini, M.A. (2009). Men's psychological transition to fatherhood: an analysis of the literature, 1989-2008. *Birth, 36*(4), 305-318.

31. Bergström, M. (2013). Depressive symptoms in new first-time fathers: Associations with age, sociodemographic characteristics, and antenatal psychological well-being. *Birth, 40*(1), 32-38.

32. Deave, T., Johnson, D., & Ingram, J. (2008). Transition to parenthood: the needs of parents in pregnancy and early parenthood. *BMC pregnancy and childbirth, 8*(1), 30.

33. Wojnar, D.M., & Katzenmeyer, A. (2014). Experiences of preconception, pregnancy, and new motherhood for lesbian nonbiological mothers. *Journal of Obstetric, Gynecologic & Neonatal Nursing, 43*(1), 50-60.

34. Larsson, A.K., & Dykes, A.K. (2009). Care during pregnancy and childbirth in Sweden: Perspectives of lesbian women. *Midwifery, 25*(6), 682-690.

35. Erlandsson, K., Linder, H., & Häggström-Nordin, E. (2010). Experiences of gay women during their partner's pregnancy and childbirth. *British journal of midwifery, 18*(2), 99-103.

36. Erlandsson, K., Linder, H., & Häggström-Nordin, E. (2010). Experiences of gay women during their partner's pregnancy and childbirth. *British journal of midwifery, 18*(2), 99-103.

37. Ziv, I., & Freund-Eschar, Y. (2015). The pregnancy experience of gay couples expecting a child through overseas surrogacy. *The Family Journal, 23*(2), 158-166.

38. Greenfeld, D.A., & Seli, E. (2011). Gay men choosing parenthood through assisted reproduction: medical and psychosocial considerations. *Fertility and sterility, 95*(1), 225-229.

39. Light, A.D., Obedin-Maliver, J., Sevelius, J.M., & Kerns, J.L. (2014). Transgender men who experienced pregnancy after female-to-male gender transitioning. *Obstetrics & Gynecology, 124*(6), 1120-1127.

40. Obedin-Maliver, J., & Makadon, H.J. (2016). Transgender men and pregnancy. *Obstetric medicine, 9*(1), 4-8.

41. Hoffkling, A., Obedin-Maliver, J., & Sevelius, J. (2017). From erasure to opportunity: a qualitative study of the experiences of transgender men around pregnancy and recommendations for providers. *BMC pregnancy and childbirth, 17*(2), 332.

42. Tavoli, Z., Mohammadi, M., Tavoli, A., Moini, A., Effatpanah, M., Khedmat, L., & Montazeri, A. (2018). Quality of life and psychological distress in women with recurrent miscarriage: a comparative study. *Health and quality of life outcomes, 16*(1), 150.

43. Brier, N. (2004). Anxiety after miscarriage: a review of the empirical literature and implications for clinical practice. *Birth, 31*(2), 138-142.

44. Rich, D. (2018). Psychological Impact of Pregnancy Loss: Best Practice for Obstetric Providers. *Clinical obstetrics and gynecology, 61*(3), 628-636.

45. Simpson, C., Lee, P., & Lionel, J. (2015). The Effect of Bereavement Counseling On Women with Psychological Problems Associated with Late Pregnancy Loss. *Journal of Asian Midwives (JAM), 2*(2), 5-20.

46. Fenstermacher, K.H., & Hupcey, J.E. (2019). Support for Young Black Urban Women After Perinatal Loss. *MCN: The American Journal of Maternal/Child Nursing*,

44(1), 13-19.

47. Adolfsson, A., Arbhede, E., Marklund, E., Larsson, P.G.O., & Berg, M. (2015). Miscarriage—Evidence Based Information for the Web and Its Development Procedure. *Advances in sexual medicine*, *5*(04), 89.

48. Van, P., Cage, T., & Shannon, M. (2004). Big dreams, little sleep: dreams during pregnancy after prior pregnancy loss. *Holistic Nursing Practice*, *18*(6), 284-292.

49. Beebe, K.R., Gay, C.L., Richoux, S.E., & Lee, K.A. (2017). Symptom experience in late pregnancy. *Journal of Obstetric, Gynecologic & Neonatal Nursing*, *46*(4), 508-520.

50. Man, G.C.W., Zhang, T., Chen, X., Wang, J., Wu, F., Liu, Y., ... & Li, T. C. (2017). The regulations and role of circadian clock and melatonin in uterine receptivity and pregnancy—an immunological perspective. *American Journal of Reproductive Immunology*, *78*(2), e12715.

51. Agarwal, A., Gupta, S., & Sharma, R. K. (2005). Role of oxidative stress in female reproduction. *Reproductive biology and endocrinology*, *3*(1), 28.

52. Mark, P.J., Crew, R.C., Wharfe, M.D., & Waddell, B.J. (2017). Rhythmic Three-Part Harmony: the complex interaction of maternal, placental and fetal circadian systems. *Journal of biological rhythms*, *32*(6), 534-549.

53. Gallaher, K.G.H., Slyepchenko, A., Frey, B.N., Urstad, K., & Dørheim, S.K. (2018). The role of circadian rhythms in postpartum sleep and mood. *Sleep medicine clinics*, *13*(3), 359-374.

54. Hux, V.J., Roberts, J.M., & Okun, M.L. (2017). Allostatic load in early pregnancy is associated with poor sleep quality. *Sleep medicine*, *33*, 85-90.

55. Hashmi, A.M., Bhatia, S.K., Bhatia, S.K., & Khawaja, I.S. (2016). Insomnia during pregnancy: diagnosis and rational interventions. *Pakistan journal of medical sciences*, *32*(4), 1030.

56. Ferini-Strambi, L., & Manconi, M. (2016). 20 Restless Legs Syndrome in Pregnancy. *Neurological Disease and Therapy*, 239.

57. Morong, S., Hermsen, B., & de Vries, N. (2015). Sleep position and pregnancy. In *Positional Therapy in Obstructive Sleep Apnea* (pp. 163-173). Springer, Cham.

58. Venkata, C., & Venkateshiah, S.B. (2009). Sleep-disordered breathing during pregnancy. *The Journal of the American Board of Family Medicine*, *22*(2), 158-168.

59. Loutzenhiser, L., McAuslan, P., & Sharpe, D.P. (2015). The trajectory of maternal and paternal fatigue and factors associated with fatigue across the transition to parenthood. *Clinical Psychologist*, *19*(1), 15-27.

60. Sarberg, M., Bladh, M., Svanborg, E., & Josefsson, A. (2016). Postpartum depressive symptoms and its association to daytime sleepiness and restless legs during pregnancy. *BMC pregnancy and childbirth*, *16*(1), 137.

61. Bergbom, I., Modh, C., Lundgren, I., & Lindwall, L. (2017). First-time pregnant women's experiences of their body in early pregnancy. *Scandinavian journal of caring sciences*, *31*(3), 579-586.

62. Miller, L.J. (2016). Psychological, Behavioral, and Cognitive Changes During Pregnancy and the Postpartum Period. In *The Oxford Handbook of Perinatal Psychology*.

63. Morong, S., Hermsen, B., & de Vries, N. (2015). Sleep position and pregnancy. In

Positional Therapy in Obstructive Sleep Apnea (pp. 163-173). Springer, Cham.

64. Body, C., & Christie, J.A. (2016). Gastrointestinal diseases in pregnancy: nausea, vomiting, hyperemesis gravidarum, gastroesophageal reflux disease, constipation, and diarrhea. *Gastroenterology Clinics, 45*(2), 267-283.

65. Swift, J.A., Langley-Evans, S.C., Pearce, J., Jethwa, P.H., Taylor, M.A., Avery, A., ... & Elliott-Sale, K.J. (2017). Antenatal weight management: Diet, physical activity, and gestational weight gain in early pregnancy. *Midwifery, 49*, 40-46.

66. Ward-Ritacco, C., Poudevigne, M.S., & O'Connor, P.J. (2016). Muscle strengthening exercises during pregnancy are associated with increased energy and reduced fatigue. *Journal of Psychosomatic Obstetrics & Gynecology, 37*(2), 68-72.

67. Baker, J.H., Rothenberger, S.D., Kline, C.E., & Okun, M.L. (2018). Exercise during early pregnancy is associated with greater sleep continuity. *Behavioral sleep medicine, 16*(5), 482-493.

68. Babbar, S., & Shyken, J. (2016). Yoga in pregnancy. *Clinical obstetrics and gynecology, 59*(3), 600-612.

69. Elrod, H. (2016). *The Miracle Morning: The 6 Habits That Will Transform Your Life Before 8AM: Change your life with one of the world's highest rated self-help books.* Hachette UK.

70. Toguchi, R.M. (2017). *The Winning Habits of Steve Jobs.* iUniverse.

Chapter 5: Relationships and sleep

1. Teti, D.M., Philbrook, L., Shimizu, M., Reader, J., Rhee, H.Y., McDaniel, B., ... & Jian, N. (2015). The social ecology of infant sleep. *Handbook of infant biopsychosocial development,* 359-391.

2. Troxel, W.M., Robles, T.F., Hall, M., & Buysse, D.J. (2007). Marital quality and the marital bed: Examining the covariation between relationship quality and sleep. *Sleep medicine reviews, 11*(5), 389-404.

3. Hasler, B.P., & Troxel, W.M. (2010). Couples' nighttime sleep efficiency and concordance: Evidence for bidirectional associations with daytime relationship functioning. *Psychosomatic Medicine, 72*(8), 794.

4. Lavner, J.A., & Bradbury, T.N. (2017). Protecting relationships from stress. *Current Opinion in Psychology, 13*, 11-14.

5. Kahn-Greene, E.T., Killgore, D.B., Kamimori, G.H., Balkin, T.J., & Killgore, W.D. (2007). The effects of sleep deprivation on symptoms of psychopathology in healthy adults. *Sleep medicine, 8*(3), 215-221.

6. Venn, S., Arber, S., Meadows, R., & Hislop, J. (2008). The fourth shift: exploring the gendered nature of sleep disruption among couples with children. *The British Journal of Sociology, 59*(1), 79-97.

7. Sirois, F.M., Bögels, S., & Emerson, L.M. (2019). Self-compassion Improves Parental Well-being in Response to Challenging Parenting Events. *The Journal of Psychology, 153*(3), 327-341.

8. TenHouten, W.D. (2018). From ressentiment to resentment as a tertiary emotion. *Review of European Studies, 10*(4), 1-16.

9. Leahy, R.L., & Tirch, D.D. (2008). Cognitive behavioral therapy for jealousy. *International Journal of Cognitive Therapy, 1*(1), 18-32.

10. Kahn-Greene, E.T., Killgore, D.B., Kamimori, G.H., Balkin, T.J., & Killgore, W.D. (2007). The effects of sleep deprivation on symptoms of psychopathology in healthy adults. *Sleep medicine, 8*(3), 215-221.

11. McDaniel, B.T., & Teti, D.M. (2012). Coparenting quality during the first three months after birth: The role of infant sleep quality. *Journal of Family Psychology, 26*(6), 886.

12. Hock, R.M., Timm, T.M., & Ramisch, J.L. (2012). Parenting children with autism spectrum disorders: A crucible for couple relationships. *Child & Family Social Work, 17*(4), 406-415.

13. Chung, M.R., Jo, H.Y., & Lee, S.H. (2018). Multi Group Analysis on the Structural Relationship between Spousal Support, Parenting Efficacy and Parenting Stress of Parents with Six-Month-Year Old Infants. *Korean Journal of Childcare and Education, 14*(2), 39-58.

14. Tikotzky, L. (2017). Parenting and sleep in early childhood. *Current Opinion in psychology, 15*, 118-124.

15. Teti, D.M., Cole, P.M., Cabrera, N., Goodman, S.H., & McLoyd, V.C. (2017). Supporting parents: How six decades of parenting research can inform policy and best practice.

16. Lavner, J.A., & Bradbury, T.N. (2017). Protecting relationships from stress. *Current Opinion in Psychology, 13*, 11-14.

17. Allen, T.D., & Kiburz, K.M. (2012). Trait mindfulness and work–family balance among working parents: The mediating effects of vitality and sleep quality. *Journal of vocational behavior, 80*(2), 372-379.

18. Whittingham, K. (2016). Mindfulness and transformative parenting. In *Mindfulness and Buddhist-Derived Approaches in Mental Health and Addiction* (pp. 363-390). Springer, Cham.

Chapter 6: Normal infant and child sleep

1. Akacem, L.D., Wright Jr, K.P., & LeBourgeois, M.K. (2016). Evening Light Exposure Infuences Circadian Timing In Preschool-Age Children: A Field Study. *Understanding Circadian Physiology in Early Childhood: the Role of Napping and Light at Night*, 107.

2. Biran, V., Decobert, F., Bednarek, N., Boizeau, P., Benoist, J.F., Claustrat, B., ... & Graesslin, O. (2019). Melatonin Levels in Preterm and Term Infants and Their Mothers. *International journal of molecular sciences, 20*(9), 2077.

3. Ivars, K., Nelson, N., Theodorsson, A., Theodorsson, E., Ström, J. O., & Mörelius, E. (2015). Development of salivary cortisol circadian rhythm and reference intervals in full-term infants. *PloS one, 10*(6), e0129502.

4. Simons, S.S., Beijers, R., Cillessen, A.H., & de Weerth, C. (2015). Development of the cortisol circadian rhythm in the light of stress early in life. *Psychoneuroendocrinology, 62*, 292-300.

5. Shukla, C., & Basheer, R. (2016). Metabolic signals in sleep regulation: recent insights. *Nature and science of sleep, 8*, 9.

6. Lok, R., van Koningsveld, M.J., Gordijn, M.C., Beersma, D.G., & Hut, R A. (2019). Daytime melatonin and light independently affect human alertness and body temperature. *Journal of pineal research, 67*(1), e12583.

7. Jenni, O.G., & Carskadon, M.A. (2005). Normal human sleep at different ages: Infants to adolescents. *SRS basics of sleep guide*, 11-19.

8. Fang, Z., & Rao, H. (2017). Imaging homeostatic sleep pressure and circadian rhythm in the human brain. *Journal of thoracic disease*, 9(5), E495.

9. Jenni, O.G., & LeBourgeois, M.K. (2006). Understanding sleep–wake behavior and sleep disorders in children: the value of a model. *Current Opinion in Psychiatry*, 19(3), 282.

10. Reichert, C.F., Maire, M., Gabel, V., Viola, A.U., Götz, T., Scheffler, K., ... & Salmon, E. (2017). Cognitive brain responses during circadian wake-promotion: evidence for sleep-pressure-dependent hypothalamic activations. *Scientific reports*, 7(1), 1-9.

11. Reichert, C.F., Maire, M., Gabel, V., Viola, A.U., Götz, T., Scheffler, K., ... & Salmon, E. (2017). Cognitive brain responses during circadian wake-promotion: evidence for sleep-pressure-dependent hypothalamic activations. *Scientific reports*, 7(1), 1-9.

12. Tikotzky, L., Sadeh, A., & Glickman-Gavrieli, T. (2010). Infant sleep and paternal involvement in infant caregiving during the first 6 months of life. *Journal of Pediatric Psychology*, 36(1), 36-46.

13. Jenni, O.G., & LeBourgeois, M.K. (2006). Understanding sleep–wake behavior and sleep disorders in children: the value of a model. *Current Opinion in Psychiatry*, 19(3), 282.

14. McDevitt, E.A., Alaynick, W.A., & Mednick, S.C. (2012). The effect of nap frequency on daytime sleep architecture. *Physiology & behavior*, 107(1), 40-44.

15. Leproult, R., & Van Cauter, E. (2010). Role of sleep and sleep loss in hormonal release and metabolism. In *Pediatric Neuroendocrinology* (Vol. 17, pp. 11-21). Karger Publishers.

16. Reichert, S., Arocas, O.P., & Rihel, J. (2019). The neuropeptide Galanin is required for homeostatic rebound sleep following increased neuronal activity. *Neuron*, 104(2), 370-384.

17. Grigg-Damberger, M.M. (2016). The visual scoring of sleep in infants 0 to 2 months of age. *Journal of Clinical Sleep Medicine*, 12(03), 429-445.

18. Dias, C.C., & Figueiredo, B. (2019). Sleep-wake behaviour during the first 12 months of life and associated factors: a systematic review. *Early Child Development and Care*, 1-33.

19. Lopp, S., Navidi, W., Achermann, P., LeBourgeois, M., & Diniz Behn, C. (2017). Developmental changes in ultradian sleep cycles across early childhood: preliminary insights. *Journal of biological rhythms*, 32(1), 64-74.

20. Korotchikova, I., Stevenson, N.J., Livingstone, V., Ryan, C.A., & Boylan, G.B. (2016). Sleep–wake cycle of the healthy term newborn infant in the immediate postnatal period. *Clinical Neurophysiology*, 127(4), 2095-2101.

21. Airhihenbuwa, C. O., Iwelunmor, J. I., Ezepue, C. J., Williams, N. J., & Jean-Louis, G. (2016). I sleep, because we sleep: a synthesis on the role of culture in sleep behavior research. *Sleep medicine*, 18, 67-73..

22. Ekirch, A.R. (2001). Sleep we have lost: pre-industrial slumber in the British Isles. *The American Historical Review*, 106(2), 343-386.

23. Matricciani, L., Olds, T., & Petkov, J. (2012). In search of lost sleep: Secular trends in the sleep time of school-aged children and adolescents. *Sleep Medicine Reviews*,

3(16), 203-211.

24. McKenna, J.J., Ball, H.L., & Gettler, L.T. (2007). Mother–infant cosleeping, breastfeeding and sudden infant death syndrome: what biological anthropology has discovered about normal infant sleep and pediatric sleep medicine. *American Journal of Physical Anthropology: The Official Publication of the American Association of Physical Anthropologists, 134*(S45), 133-161.

25. Blunden, S.L., Thompson, K.R., & Dawson, D. (2011). Behavioural sleep treatments and night time crying in infants: challenging the status quo. *Sleep medicine reviews, 15*(5), 327-334.

26. Daly, S.E., & Hartmann, P.E. (1995). Infant demand and milk supply. Part 2: The short-term control of milk synthesis in lactating women. *Journal of Human Lactation, 11*(1), 27-37.

27. Parslow, P.M., Harding, R., Adamson, T.M., & Horne, R.S. (2004). Effects of sleep state and postnatal age on arousal responses induced by mild hypoxia in infants. *Sleep, 27*(1), 105-109.

28. Mindell, J.A., Sadeh, A., Wiegand, B., How, T.H., & Goh, D.Y. (2010). Cross-cultural differences in infant and toddler sleep. *Sleep medicine, 11*(3), 274-280.

29. Jenni, O.G., & Carskadon, M.A. (2005). Normal human sleep at different ages: Infants to adolescents. *SRS basics of sleep guide*, 11-19.

30. Verbiest, S.B., Tully, K.P., & Stuebe, A.M. (2017). Promoting maternal and infant health in the 4th trimester. *Zero to Three, 37*(4), 34-44.

31. Tully, K.P., Stuebe, A.M., & Verbiest, S.B. (2017). The fourth trimester: a critical transition period with unmet maternal health needs. *American Journal of Obstetrics and Gynecology, 217*(1), 37-41.

32. Vasak, M., Williamson, J., Garden, J., & Zwicker, J. G. (2015). Sensory processing and sleep in typically developing infants and toddlers. *American Journal of Occupational Therapy, 69*(4), 6904220040p1-6904220040p8.

33. Shavit, Y., Friedman, I., Gal, J., & Vaknin, D. (2018). Emerging Early Childhood Inequality: On the Relationship Between Poverty, Sensory Stimulation, Child Development, and Achievement.

34. Nelson, C.A., Zeanah, C.H., & Fox, N.A. (2019). How Early Experience Shapes Human Development: The Case of Psychosocial Deprivation. *Neural plasticity, 2019*.

35. Watamura, S.E., Donzella, B., Kertes, D.A., & Gunnar, M.R. (2004). Developmental changes in baseline cortisol activity in early childhood: Relations with napping and effortful control. *Developmental Psychobiology: The Journal of the International Society for Developmental Psychobiology, 45*(3), 125-133.

36. Adams, S. M., Jones, D. R., Esmail, A., & Mitchell, E. A. (2004). What affects the age of first sleeping through the night?. *Journal of paediatrics and child health, 40*(3), 96-101.

37. Henderson, J.M., France, K.G., Owens, J.L., & Blampied, N.M. (2010). Sleeping through the night: the consolidation of self-regulated sleep across the first year of life. *Pediatrics, 126*(5), e1081.

38. Mindell, J.A., Leichman, E.S., Composto, J., Lee, C., Bhullar, B., & Walters, R.M. (2016). Development of infant and toddler sleep patterns: real-world data from a mobile

application. *Journal of Sleep Research, 25*(5), 508-516.

39. Brown, A., & Harries, V. (2015). Infant sleep and night feeding patterns during later infancy: Association with breastfeeding frequency, daytime complementary food intake, and infant weight. *Breastfeeding Medicine, 10*(5), 246-252.

40. Hysing, M., Harvey, A.G., Torgersen, L., Ystrom, E., Reichborn-Kjennerud, T., & Sivertsen, B. (2014). Trajectories and predictors of nocturnal awakenings and sleep duration in infants. *Journal of Developmental & Behavioral Pediatrics, 35*(5), 309-316.

41. Adams, S. M., Jones, D. R., Esmail, A., & Mitchell, E. A. (2004). What affects the age of first sleeping through the night?. *Journal of paediatrics and child health, 40*(3), 96-101

42. St James-Roberts, I., Roberts, M., Hovish, K., & Owen, C. (2015). Video evidence that London infants can resettle themselves back to sleep after waking in the night, as well as sleep for long periods, by 3 months of age. *Journal of Developmental and Behavioral Pediatrics, 36*(5), 324.

43. Sadeh, A., Tikotzky, L., & Scher, A. (2010). Parenting and infant sleep. *Sleep medicine reviews, 14*(2), 89-96.

44. Tikotzky, L., Sadeh, A., & Glickman-Gavrieli, T. (2010). Infant sleep and paternal involvement in infant caregiving during the first 6 months of life. *Journal of Pediatric Psychology, 36*(1), 36-46.

45. Henderson, J.M., France, K.G., Owens, J.L., & Blampied, N.M. (2010). Sleeping through the night: the consolidation of self-regulated sleep across the first year of life. *Pediatrics, 126*(5), e1081.

46. Goodlin-Jones, B.L., Burnham, M.M., Gaylor, E.E., & Anders, T.F. (2001). Night waking, sleep-wake organization, and self-soothing in the first year of life. *Journal of developmental and behavioral pediatrics: JDBP, 22*(4), 226.

47. Sadeh, A., Tikotzky, L., & Scher, A. (2010). Parenting and infant sleep. *Sleep medicine reviews, 14*(2), 89-96.

48. Magee, C.A., Gordon, R., & Caputi, P. (2014). Distinct developmental trends in sleep duration during early childhood. *Pediatrics, 133*(6), e1561-e1567.

49. Joseph, D., Chong, N.W., Shanks, M.E., Rosato, E., Taub, N.A., Petersen, S.A., ... & Wailoo, M. (2015). Getting rhythm: how do babies do it?. *Archives of Disease in Childhood-Fetal and Neonatal Edition, 100*(1), F50-F54.

50. Marcus, C.L., Brooks, L.J., Ward, S.D., Draper, K.A., Gozal, D., Halbower, A.C., ... & Shiffman, R.N. (2012). Diagnosis and management of childhood obstructive sleep apnea syndrome. *Pediatrics, 130*(3), e714-e755.

51. Marcus, C.L., Traylor, J., Gallagher, P.R., Brooks, L.J., Huang, J., Koren, D., ... & Tapia, I.E. (2014). Prevalence of periodic limb movements during sleep in normal children. *Sleep, 37*(8), 1349-1352.

52. Coffey, J. (2006). Parenting a child with chronic illness: a metasynthesis. *Pediatric Nursing, 32*, 9.

53. Lewis-Jones, S. (2006). Quality of life and childhood atopic dermatitis: the misery of living with childhood eczema. *International Journal of Clinical Practice, 60*(8), 984-992.

54. Tauman, R., Levine, A., Avni, H., Nehama, H., Greenfeld, M., & Sivan, Y. (2011).

Coexistence of sleep and feeding disturbances in young children. *Pediatrics, 127*(3), e615-e621.

55. von Kries, R., Kalies, H., & Papousek, M. (2006). Excessive Crying Beyond 3 Months May Herald Other Features of Multiple Regulatory Problems. *Archives of Pediatric and Adolescent Medicine, 160,* 508-511

56. Watson-Genna, C. (2013). *Supporting Sucking Skills in Breastfeeding Infants.* New York: Jones and Bartlett Learning.

57. Hazelbaker, A. (2010). *Tongue-Tie. Morphogenesis, Impact, Assessment and Treatment.* Ohio: Aiden and Eva Press.

58. Colson, E. R., Willinger, M., Rybin, D., Heeren, T., Smith, L. A., Lister, G., & Corwin, M. J. (2013). Trends and factors associated with infant bed sharing, 1993-2010: the National Infant Sleep Position Study. *JAMA pediatrics, 167*(11), 1032-1037.

59. Ball, H.L. (2017). The Atlantic divide: Contrasting UK and US recommendations on cosleeping and bed-sharing. *Journal of Human Lactation, 33*(4), 765-769.

60. Ward, T.C.S. (2015). Reasons for mother–infant bed-sharing: A systematic narrative synthesis of the literature and implications for future research. *Maternal and child health journal, 19*(3), 675-690.

61. Ball, H.L., Howel, D., Bryant, A., Best, E., Russell, C., & Ward-Platt, M. (2016). Bed-sharing by breastfeeding mothers: who bed-shares and what is the relationship with breastfeeding duration?. *Acta Paediatrica, 105*(6), 628-634.

62. Tomori, C., Palmquist, A.E., & Dowling, S. (2016). Contested moral landscapes: Negotiating breastfeeding stigma in breastmilk sharing, nighttime breastfeeding, and long-term breastfeeding in the US and the UK. *Social Science & Medicine, 168,* 178-185.

63. McKenna, J.J., & Gettler, L.T. (2016). There is no such thing as infant sleep, there is no such thing as breastfeeding, there is only breastsleeping. *Acta Paediatrica, 105*(1), 17-21.

64. Blair, P.S., Heron, J., & Fleming, P.J. (2010). Relationship between bed sharing and breastfeeding: longitudinal, population-based analysis. *Pediatrics, 126*(5), e1119-e1126.

65. Jenni, O.G., Fuhrer, H.Z., Iglowstein, I., Molinari, L., & Largo, R.H. (2005). A longitudinal study of bed sharing and sleep problems among Swiss children in the first 10 years of life. *Pediatrics, 115*(1 Suppl), 233-240.

66. Task Force on Sudden Infant Death Syndrome. (2016). SIDS and other sleep-related infant deaths: Updated 2016 recommendations for a safe infant sleeping environment. *Pediatrics, 138*(5), e20162938.

67. NICE Postnatal Care Guidance. 2014. Recommendation 1.4.47: Co-sleeping and Sudden Infant Death Syndrome https://www.nice.org.uk/guidance/cg37/chapter/1-recommendations#maintaining-infanthealth

68. Ball, H.L., Moya, E., Fairley, L., Westman, J., Oddie, S., & Wright, J. (2012). Bed-and sofa-sharing practices in a UK biethnic population. *Pediatrics, 129*(3), e673-e681.

69. Blair, P.S., Sidebotham, P., Pease, A., & Fleming, P.J. (2014). Bed-sharing in the absence of hazardous circumstances: is there a risk of sudden infant death syndrome? An analysis from two case-control studies conducted in the UK. *PLoS One, 9*(9), e107799.

70. Mileva-Seitz, V.R., Bakermans-Kranenburg, M.J., Battaini, C., & Luijk, M.P. (2017). Parent-child bed-sharing: the good, the bad, and the burden of evidence. *Sleep Medicine Reviews, 32*, 4-27.

71. Vennemann, M.M., Hense, H.W., Bajanowski, T., Blair, P.S., Complojer, C., Moon, R.Y., & Kiechl-Kohlendorfer, U. (2012). Bed sharing and the risk of sudden infant death syndrome: can we resolve the debate?. *The Journal of pediatrics, 160*(1), 44-48.

72. Carpenter, R., McGarvey, C., Mitchell, E.A., Tappin, D.M., Vennemann, M.M., Smuk, M., & Carpenter, J.R. (2013). Bed sharing when parents do not smoke: is there a risk of SIDS? An individual level analysis of five major case–control studies. *BMJ open, 3*(5), e002299.

73. Ball, H.L. (2015). Empowering families to make informed choices about sleep safety. *British Journal of Midwifery., 23*(3), 164-165.

Chapter 7: Naps

1. McDevitt, E.A., Alaynick, W.A., & Mednick, S.C. (2012). The effect of nap frequency on daytime sleep architecture. *Physiology & behavior, 107*(1), 40-44.

2. Anderson, G., Vaillancourt, C., Maes, M., & Reiter, R.J. (2016). Breast Feeding and Melatonin: Implications for Improving Perinatal Health. *Journal of Breastfeeding Biology, 1*(1), 8.

3. Salzarulo, P., & Fagioli, I. (1992). Sleep-wake rhythms and sleep structure in the first year of life. In *Why we nap* (pp. 50-57). Birkhäuser, Boston, MA.

4. Gribbin, C.E., Watamura, S.E., Cairns, A., Harsh, J.R., & LeBourgeois, M.K. (2012). The cortisol awakening response (CAR) in 2-to 4-year-old children: Effects of acute nighttime sleep restriction, wake time, and daytime napping. *Developmental psychobiology, 54*(4), 412-422.

5. Endo, T., Roth, C., Landolt, H.P., Werth, E., Aeschbach, D., Achermann, P., & Borbély, A.A. (1998). Selective REM sleep deprivation in humans: effects on sleep and sleep EEG. *American Journal of Physiology-Regulatory, Integrative and Comparative Physiology, 274*(4), R1186-R1194.

6. Buckley, T.M., & Schatzberg, A.F. (2005). On the interactions of the hypothalamic-pituitary-adrenal (HPA) axis and sleep: normal HPA axis activity and circadian rhythm, exemplary sleep disorders. *The Journal of Clinical Endocrinology & Metabolism, 90*(5), 3106-3114.

7. Elmenhorst, E.M., Elmenhorst, D., Luks, N., Maass, H., Vejvoda, M., & Samel, A. (2008). Partial sleep deprivation: impact on the architecture and quality of sleep. *Sleep medicine, 9*(8), 840-850.

8. Aeschbach, D. (2011). REM-sleep regulation: circadian, homeostatic, and non-REM sleep-dependent determinants. *Rapid Eye Movement Sleep: Regulation and Function. Cambridge University Press, Cambridge*, 80-88.

9. Muto, V., Jaspar, M., Meyer, C., Kussé, C., Chellappa, S. L., Degueldre, C., ... & Archer, S.N. (2016). Local modulation of human brain responses by circadian rhythmicity and sleep debt. *Science, 353*(6300), 687-690.

10. Galland, B.C., Taylor, B.J., Elder, D.E., & Herbison, P. (2012). Normal sleep patterns in infants and children: a systematic review of observational studies. *Sleep medicine reviews, 16*(3), 213-222.

11. Hirshkowitz, M., Whiton, K., Albert, S. M., Alessi, C., Bruni, O., DonCarlos, L., ... & Neubauer, D.N. (2015). National Sleep Foundation's sleep time duration recommendations: methodology and results summary. *Sleep health, 1*(1), 40-43.

12. Ohayon, M., Wickwire, E.M., Hirshkowitz, M., Albert, S.M., Avidan, A., Daly, F.J., ... & Hazen, N. (2017). National Sleep Foundation's sleep quality recommendations: first report. *Sleep Health, 3*(1), 6-19.

13. Iglowstein, I., Jenni, O.G., Molinari, L., & Largo, R.H. (2003). Sleep duration from infancy to adolescence: reference values and generational trends. *Pediatrics-Springfield, 111*(3), 302-307.

14. Larson, M.C., Gunnar, M.R., & Hertsgaard, L. (1991). The effects of morning naps, car trips, and maternal separation on adrenocortical activity in human infants. *Child development, 62*(2), 362-372.

15. Byars, K.C., Yolton, K., Rausch, J., Lanphear, B., & Beebe, D.W. (2012). Prevalence, patterns, and persistence of sleep problems in the first 3 years of life. *Pediatrics, 129*(2), e276.

16. McDevitt, E.A., Alaynick, W.A., & Mednick, S.C. (2012). The effect of nap frequency on daytime sleep architecture. *Physiology & behavior, 107*(1), 40-44.

17. Skuladottir, A., Thome, M., & Ramel, A. (2005). Improving day and night sleep problems in infants by changing day time sleep rhythm: a single group before and after study. *International Journal of nursing studies, 42*(8), 843-850.

18. Fukuda, K., & Sakashita, Y. (2002). Sleeping pattern of kindergartners and nursery school children: function of daytime nap. *Perceptual and motor skills, 94*(1), 219-228.

19. Thorpe, K., Staton, S., Sawyer, E., Pattinson, C., Haden, C., & Smith, S. (2015). Napping, development and health from 0 to 5 years: a systematic review. *Archives of Disease in Childhood, 100*(7), 615-622.

20. Anuntaseree, W., Mo-Suwan, L., Vasiknanonte, P., Kuasirikul, S., & Choprapawan, C. (2008). Night waking in Thai infants at 3 months of age: association between parental practices and infant sleep. *Sleep Medicine, 9*(5), 564-571.

Chapter 8: Night feeds

1. Mindell, J.A., & Owens, J.A. (2015). *A clinical guide to pediatric sleep: diagnosis and management of sleep problems.* Lippincott Williams & Wilkins.

2. Brown, A., & Harries, V. (2015). Infant sleep and night feeding patterns during later infancy: Association with breastfeeding frequency, daytime complementary food intake, and infant weight. *Breastfeeding Medicine, 10*(5), 246-252.

3. Hysing, M., Harvey, A. G., Torgersen, L., Ystrom, E., Reichborn-Kjennerud, T., & Sivertsen, B. (2014). Trajectories and predictors of nocturnal awakenings and sleep duration in infants. *Journal of Developmental & Behavioral Pediatrics, 35*(5), 309-316.

4. Brown, A., & Harries, V. (2015). Infant sleep and night feeding patterns during later infancy: Association with breastfeeding frequency, daytime complementary food intake, and infant weight. *Breastfeeding Medicine, 10*(5), 246-252.

5. Hysing, M., Harvey, A. G., Torgersen, L., Ystrom, E., Reichborn-Kjennerud, T., & Sivertsen, B. (2014). Trajectories and predictors of nocturnal awakenings and sleep

duration in infants. *Journal of Developmental & Behavioral Pediatrics, 35*(5), 309-316.

6. Weinraub, M., Bender, R.H., Friedman, S.L., Susman, E.J., Knoke, B., Bradley, R., ... & Williams, J. (2012). Patterns of developmental change in infants' nighttime sleep awakenings from 6 through 36 months of age. *Developmental psychology, 48*(6), 1511-1528.

7. Hall, W.A., Saunders, R.A., Clauson, M., Carty, E.M. and Janssen, P.A., 2006. Effects of an intervention aimed at reducing night waking and signaling in 6-to 12-month-old infants. *Behavioral Sleep Medicine, 4*(4), pp.242-261.

8. Kapás, L. (2010). Metabolic signals in sleep regulation: the role of cholecystokinin. *Doctor Thesis.*

9. Shukla, C., & Basheer, R. (2016). Metabolic signals in sleep regulation: recent insights. *Nature and science of sleep, 8*, 9.

10. Cordeira, J., & Rios, M. (2011). Weighing in the role of BDNF in the central control of eating behavior. *Molecular neurobiology, 44*(3), 441-448.

11. Müller, T.D., Nogueiras, R., Andermann, M.L., Andrews, Z.B., Anker, S.D., Argente, J., ... & Casanueva, F.F. (2015). Ghrelin. *Molecular metabolism, 4*(6), 437-460.

12. Rodgers, R.J., Ishii, Y., Halford, J.C.G., & Blundell, J.E. (2002). Orexins and appetite regulation. *Neuropeptides, 36*(5), 303-325.

13. Venner, A., Karnani, M.M., Gonzalez, J.A., Jensen, L.T., Fugger, L., & Burdakov, D. (2011). Orexin neurons as conditional glucosensors: paradoxical regulation of sugar sensing by intracellular fuels. *The Journal of Physiology, 589*(23), 5701-5708.

14. Whittingham, K., & Douglas, P. (2014). Optimizing parent-infant sleep from birth to 6 months: A new paradigm. *Infant mental health journal, 35*(6), 614-623.

15. Goel, N., Stunkard, A J., Rogers, N.L., Van Dongen, H.P., Allison, K.C., O'Reardon, J.P., ... & Dinges, D.F. (2009). Circadian rhythm profiles in women with night eating syndrome. *Journal of biological rhythms, 24*(1), 85-94.

16. Kim, T.W., Jeong, J.H., & Hong, S.C. (2015). The impact of sleep and circadian disturbance on hormones and metabolism. *International Journal of Endocrinology, 2015.*

17. Wehrens, S.M., Christou, S., Isherwood, C., Middleton, B., Gibbs, M.A., Archer, S.N., ... & Johnston, J.D. (2017). Meal timing regulates the human circadian system. *Current Biology, 27*(12), 1768-1775.

18. Wehrens, S.M., Christou, S., Isherwood, C., Middleton, B., Gibbs, M.A., Archer, S.N., ... & Johnston, J.D. (2017). Meal timing regulates the human circadian system. *Current Biology, 27*(12), 1768-1775.

19. Taheri, S., Lin, L., Austin, D., Young, T., & Mignot, E. (2004). Short sleep duration is associated with reduced leptin, elevated ghrelin, and increased body mass index. *PLoS medicine, 1*(3), e62.

20. Hart, C.N., Carskadon, M.A., Considine, R.V., Fava, J.L., Lawton, J., Raynor, H.A., ... & Wing, R. (2013). Changes in children's sleep duration on food intake, weight, and leptin. *Pediatrics, 132*(6), e1473-e1480.

21. Adair, R., Bauchner, H., Philipp, B., Levenson, S., & Zuckerman, B. (1991). Night waking during infancy: role of parental presence at bedtime. *Pediatrics, 87*(4), 500-504.

22. Anders, T.F., Halpern, L.F., & Hua, J. (1992). Sleeping through the night: a developmental perspective. *Pediatrics*, *90*(4), 554-560.

23. Goodlin-Jones, B.L., Burnham, M.M., Gaylor, E.E., & Anders, T.F. (2001). Night waking, sleep-wake organization, and self-soothing in the first year of life. *Journal of developmental and behavioral pediatrics: JDBP*, *22*(4), 226.

24. St James-Roberts, I., Roberts, M., Hovish, K., & Owen, C. (2015). Video evidence that London infants can resettle themselves back to sleep after waking in the night, as well as sleep for long periods, by 3 months of age. *Journal of Developmental and Behavioral Pediatrics*, *36*(5), 324.

25. Paul, I.M., Savage, J.S., Anzman-Frasca, S., Marini, M.E., Mindell, J.A., & Birch, L.L. (2016). INSIGHT responsive parenting intervention and infant sleep. *Pediatrics*, *138*(1).

26. Sette, S., Baumgartner, E., Ferri, R., & Bruni, O. (2017). Predictors of sleep disturbances in the first year of life: a longitudinal study. *Sleep medicine*, *36*, 78-85.

27. Ramamurthy, M.B., Sekartini, R., Ruangdaraganon, N., Huynh, D.H.T., Sadeh, A., & Mindell, J.A. (2012). Effect of current breastfeeding on sleep patterns in infants from Asia-Pacific region. *Journal of paediatrics and child health*, *48*(8), 669-674.

28. Galland, B.C., Sayers, R.M., Cameron, S.L., Gray, A.R., Heath, A.L.M., Lawrence, J.A., ... & Taylor, R.W. (2017). Anticipatory guidance to prevent infant sleep problems within a randomised controlled trial: infant, maternal and partner outcomes at 6 months of age. *BMJ open*, *7*(5), e014908.

29. Whittingham, K., & Douglas, P. (2014). Optimizing parent–infant sleep from birth to 6 months: A new paradigm. *Infant mental health journal*, *35*(6), 614-623.

30. Pinilla, T., & Birch, L.L. (1993). Help Me Make It Through the Night: Behavioural Entrainment Breast-Fed Infants' Sleep Patterns. *Pediatrics*, *91*(2), 436-444.

Chapter 9: Why not leave them to cry?

1. Oster, E. (2019) *Cribsheet: A Data-Driven Guide to Better, More Relaxed Parenting from Birth to Preschool*. Penguin: London.

2. Canapari, C. (2019) *It's Never Too Late To Sleep Train*. Rodale: Emmaus.

3. Asmussen, K., & Brims, L. (2018) What works to enhance the effectiveness of the Healthy Child Program: An evidence update. EIF Report. Available online: www.eif.org.uk/report/what-works-to-enhance-the-effectiveness-of-the-healthy-child-programme-an-evidence-update

4. Hiscock, H., & Davey, M.J. (2018). Sleep disorders in infants and children. *Journal of Paediatrics and Child Health*, *54*(9), 941-944.

5. Sadeh, A., Juda-Hanael, M., Livne-Karp, E., Kahn, M., Tikotzky, L., Anders, T. F., ... & Sivan, Y. (2016). Low parental tolerance for infant crying: an underlying factor in infant sleep problems?. *Journal of Sleep Research*, *25*(5), 501-507.

6. Gradisar, M., Jackson, K., Spurrier, N.J., Gibson, J., Whitham, J., Williams, A.S., ... & Kennaway, D.J. (2016). Behavioral interventions for infant sleep problems: a randomized controlled trial. *Pediatrics*, *137*(6), e20151486.

7. Hiscock, H., Bayer, J.K., Hampton, A., Ukoumunne, O.C., & Wake, M. (2008). Long-term mother and child mental health effects of a population-based infant sleep intervention: cluster-randomized, controlled trial. *Pediatrics*, *122*(3), e621-e627.

8. Price, A.M., Wake, M., Ukoumunne, O.C., & Hiscock, H. (2012). Five-year follow-up of harms and benefits of behavioral infant sleep intervention: randomized trial. *Pediatrics*, *130*(4), 643-651.

9. Hiscock, H., Bayer, J.K., Hampton, A., Ukoumunne, O.C., & Wake, M. (2008). Long-term mother and child mental health effects of a population-based infant sleep intervention: cluster-randomized, controlled trial. *Pediatrics*, *122*(3), e621-e627.

10. Price, A.M., Wake, M., Ukoumunne, O.C., & Hiscock, H. (2012). Five-year follow-up of harms and benefits of behavioral infant sleep intervention: randomized trial. *Pediatrics*, *130*(4), 643-651.

11. Gradisar, M., Jackson, K., Spurrier, N.J., Gibson, J., Whitham, J., Williams, A.S., ... & Kennaway, D.J. (2016). Behavioral interventions for infant sleep problems: a randomized controlled trial. *Pediatrics*, *137*(6), e20151486.

12. Ainsworth, M.S., & Bowlby, J. (1991). An ethological approach to personality development. *American Psychologist*, *46*(4), 333.

13. Middlemiss, W., Granger, D.A., Goldberg, W.A., & Nathans, L. (2012). Asynchrony of mother–infant hypothalamic-pituitary-adrenal axis activity following extinction of infant crying responses induced during the transition to sleep. *Early human development*, *88*(4), 227-232.

14. Douglas, P.S., & Hill, P.S. (2013). Behavioral sleep interventions in the first six months of life do not improve outcomes for mothers or infants: a systematic review. *Journal of Developmental & Behavioral Pediatrics*, *34*(7), 497-507.

15. McLaughlin, K.A., Sheridan, M.A., Tibu, F., Fox, N.A., Zeanah, C.H., & Nelson, C.A. (2015). Causal effects of the early caregiving environment on development of stress response systems in children. *Proceedings of the National Academy of Sciences*, *112*(18), 5637-5642.

16. Scher, A. (2001). Attachment and sleep: A study of night waking in 12-month-old infants. *Developmental Psychobiology: The Journal of the International Society for Developmental Psychobiology*, *38*(4), 274-285.

17. Teti, D.M., Kim, B.R., Mayer, G., Countermine, M. Maternal emotional availability at bedtime predicts infant sleep quality. *Journal of Family Psychology*. (2010);24:307-315.

18. Bélanger, M.È., Bernier, A., Simard, V., Bordeleau, S., & Carrier, J. (2015). VIII. Attachment and sleep among toddlers: Disentangling attachment security and dependency. *Monographs of the Society for Research in Child Development*, *80*(1), 125-140.

19. Pennestri, M.H., Moss, E., O'Donnell, K., Lecompte, V., Bouvette-Turcot, A.A., Atkinson, L., ... & Gaudreau, H. (2015). Establishment and consolidation of the sleep-wake cycle as a function of attachment pattern. *Attachment & human development*, *17*(1), 23-42.

20. McLaughlin, K.A., Sheridan, M.A., Tibu, F., Fox, N.A., Zeanah, C.H., & Nelson, C.A. (2015). Causal effects of the early caregiving environment on development of stress response systems in children. *Proceedings of the National Academy of Sciences*, *112*(18), 5637-5642.

21. Francis, D.D., & Meaney, M.J. (1999). Maternal care and the development of stress responses. *Current opinion in neurobiology*, *9*(1), 128-134.

22. Ivars, K., Nelson, N., Theodorsson, A., Theodorsson, E., Ström, J.O., & Mörelius, E. (2015). Development of salivary cortisol circadian rhythm and reference intervals in full-term infants. *PloS one, 10*(6), e0129502.

23. Simons, S.S., Beijers, R., Cillessen, A.H., & de Weerth, C. (2015). Development of the cortisol circadian rhythm in the light of stress early in life. *Psychoneuroendocrinology, 62*, 292-300.

24. Bailey, S.L., & Heitkemper, M.M. (2001). Circadian rhythmicity of cortisol and body temperature: morningness-eveningness effects. *Chronobiology International, 18*(2), 249-261.

25. Randler, C., Faßl, C., & Kalb, N. (2017). From Lark to Owl: developmental changes in morningness-eveningness from new-borns to early adulthood. *Scientific Reports, 7*, 45874.

26. Simons, S.S., Cillessen, A.H., & de Weerth, C. (2017). Associations between circadian and stress response cortisol in children. *Stress, 20*(1), 69-75.

27. Simons, S.S., Cillessen, A.H., & de Weerth, C. (2017). Associations between circadian and stress response cortisol in children. *Stress, 20*(1), 69-75.

28. Fazio, L.K., Brashier, N.M., Payne, B.K., & Marsh, E.J. (2015). Knowledge does not protect against illusory truth. *Journal of Experimental Psychology: General, 144*(5), 993.

29. Oster, E. (2019) *Cribsheet: A Data-Driven Guide to Better, More Relaxed Parenting from Birth to Preschool*. Penguin: London.

30. Canapari, C. (2019) *It's Never Too Late To Sleep Train*. Rodale: Emmaus.

31. Asmussen, K., & Brims, L. (2018) What works to enhance the effectiveness of the Healthy Child Program: An evidence update. EIF Report. Available online: www.eif.org.uk/report/what-works-to-enhance-the-effectiveness-of-the-healthy-child-programme-an-evidence-update

32. De Jong, A.R. (2016). Domestic violence, children, and toxic stress. *Widener L. Rev., 22*, 201.

33. Voltaire, S.T., & Teti, D.M. (2018). Early nighttime parental interventions and infant sleep regulation across the first year. *Sleep Medicine, 52*, 107-115.

34. De Jong, A.R. (2016). Domestic violence, children, and toxic stress. *Widener L. Rev., 22*, 201.

35. Teti, D.M., Cole, P.M., Cabrera, N., Goodman, S.H., & McLoyd, V.C. (2017). Supporting parents: How six decades of parenting research can inform policy and best practice.

Chapter 10: How to gently optimise your child's sleep

1. Blunden, S.L., Thompson, K.R., & Dawson, D. (2011). Behavioural sleep treatments and night time crying in infants: challenging the status quo. *Sleep medicine reviews, 15*(5), 327-334.

2. Field, T. (2017). Infant sleep problems and interventions: A review. *Infant Behavior and Development, 47*, 40-53.

3. Harries, V., & Brown, A. (2017). The association between use of infant parenting books that promote strict routines, and maternal depression, self-efficacy, and parenting confidence. *Early Child Development and Care*, 1-12.

4. Scher, A. (2001). Attachment and sleep: A study of night waking in 12-month-old infants. *Developmental Psychobiology: The Journal of the International Society for Developmental Psychobiology, 38*(4), 274-285.

5. Bélanger, M.È., Bernier, A., Simard, V., Bordeleau, S., & Carrier, J. (2015). VIII. Attachment and sleep among toddlers: Disentangling attachment security and dependency. *Monographs of the Society for Research in Child Development, 80*(1), 125-140.

6. Pennestri, M.H., Moss, E., O'Donnell, K., Lecompte, V., Bouvette-Turcot, A.A., Atkinson, L., ... & Gaudreau, H. (2015). Establishment and consolidation of the sleep-wake cycle as a function of attachment pattern. *Attachment & human development, 17*(1), 23-42.

7. Middlemiss, W., Stevens, H., Ridgway, L., McDonald, S., & Koussa, M. (2017). Response-based sleep intervention: Helping infants sleep without making them cry. *Early Human Development, 108*, 49-57.

8. Teti, D.M., Kim, B.R., Mayer, G., Countermine, M. Maternal emotional availability at bedtime predicts infant sleep quality. *Journal of Family Psychology.* (2010);24:307-315.

9. Philbrook, L.E., & Teti, D.M. (2016). Bidirectional associations between bedtime parenting and infant sleep: Parenting quality, parenting practices, and their interaction. *Journal of Family Psychology, 30*(4), 431.

10. Jian, N., & Teti, D.M. (2016). Emotional availability at bedtime, infant temperament, and infant sleep development from one to six months. *Sleep medicine, 23*, 49-58.

11. Bedrosian, T.A., & Nelson, R.J. (2017). Timing of light exposure affects mood and brain circuits. *Translational Psychiatry, 7*(1), e1017.

12. Mindell, J.A., Li, A.M., Sadeh, A., Kwon, R., & Goh, D.Y. (2015). Bedtime routines for young children: a dose-dependent association with sleep outcomes. *Sleep, 38*(5), 717-722.

13. Teti, D.M., Cole, P.M., Cabrera, N., Goodman, S.H., & McLoyd, V.C. (2017). Supporting parents: How six decades of parenting research can inform policy and best practice.

14. Tikotzky, L. (2017). Parenting and sleep in early childhood. *Current Opinion in psychology, 15*, 118-124.

15. El-Sheikh, M., & Kelly, R.J. (2017). Family functioning and children's sleep. *Child Development Perspectives, 11*(4), 264-269.

16. Teti, D.M., Cole, P.M., Cabrera, N., Goodman, S.H., & McLoyd, V.C. (2017). Supporting parents: How six decades of parenting research can inform policy and best practice.

17. Staples, A.D., Bates, J.E., & Petersen, I.T. (2015). Ix. Bedtime routines in early childhood: Prevalence, consistency, and associations with nighttime sleep. *Monographs of the Society for Research in Child Development, 80*(1), 141-159.

18. Mindell, J.A., Li, A.M., Sadeh, A., Kwon, R., & Goh, D.Y. (2015). Bedtime routines for young children: a dose-dependent association with sleep outcomes. *Sleep, 38*(5), 717-722.

19. Prochazkova, E., & Kret, M.E. (2017). Connecting minds and sharing emotions through mimicry: A neurocognitive model of emotional contagion. *Neuroscience & Biobehavioral Reviews, 80*, 99-114.

20. Cacioppo, J.T., Tassinary, L.G., & Berntson, G.G. (2000). Psychophysiological science.

Handbook of psychophysiology, 2, 3-23.

21. Chartrand, T.L., & Van Baaren, R. (2009). Human mimicry. *Advances in experimental social psychology, 41*, 219-274.

22. Telles, S., Sharma, S.K., & Balkrishna, A. (2014). Blood pressure and heart rate variability during yoga-based alternate nostril breathing practice and breath awareness. *Medical Science Monitor Basic Research, 20*, 184.

23. Teti, D.M., & Crosby, B. (2012). Maternal depressive symptoms, dysfunctional cognitions, and infant night waking: The role of maternal nighttime behavior. *Child Development, 83*(3), 939-953.

24. Whittingham, K., & Douglas, P. (2014). Optimizing parent–infant sleep from birth to 6 months: A new paradigm. *Infant Mental Health Journal, 35*(6), 614-623.

25. Kuypers, L. (2011). *The Zones of Regulation*. San Jose: Think Social Publishing.

26. Jenni, O.G., & LeBourgeois, M.K. (2006). Understanding sleep–wake behavior and sleep disorders in children: the value of a model. *Current Opinion in Psychiatry, 19*(3), 282.

27. Carey, W.B. (1974). Night waking and temperament in infancy. *The Journal of Pediatrics, 84*(5), 756-758.

28. Sadeh, A. (1994). Assessment of intervention for infant night waking: parental reports and activity-based home monitoring. *Journal of Consulting and Clinical Psychology, 62*(1), 63.

29. De Marcas, G.S., Soffer-Dudek, N., Dollberg, S., Bar-Haim, Y., & Sadeh, A. (2015). IV. Reactivity and sleep in infants: a longitudinal objective assessment. *Monographs of the Society for Research in Child Development, 80*(1), 49-69.

30. Thorpe, K., Staton, S., Sawyer, E., Pattinson, C., Haden, C., & Smith, S. (2015). Napping, development and health from 0 to 5 years: a systematic review. *Archives of Disease in Childhood, 100*(7), 615-622.

31. Bernier, A., Tétreault, É., Bélanger, M.È., & Carrier, J. (2017). Paternal involvement and child sleep: A look beyond infancy. *International Journal of Behavioral Development, 41*(6), 714-722.

32. Rhoades, K.A., Leve, L.D., Harold, G.T., Mannering, A.M., Neiderhiser, J.M., Shaw, D.S., ... & Reiss, D. (2012). Marital hostility and child sleep problems: Direct and indirect associations via hostile parenting. *Journal of Family Psychology, 26*(4), 488.

33. Philbrook, L.E., & Teti, D.M. (2016). Bidirectional associations between bedtime parenting and infant sleep: Parenting quality, parenting practices, and their interaction. *Journal of Family Psychology, 30*(4), 431.

34. Gertner, S., Greenbaum, C.W., Sadeh, A., Dolfin, Z., Sirota, L., & Ben-Nun, Y. (2002). Sleep–wake patterns in preterm infants and 6 month's home environment: implications for early cognitive development. *Early Human Development, 68*(2), 93-102.

35. Whittingham, K. (2016). Mindfulness and transformative parenting. In *Mindfulness and Buddhist-Derived Approaches in Mental Health and Addiction* (pp. 363-390). Springer, Cham.

36. Schneider, N., Mutungi, G., & Cubero, J. (2018). Diet and nutrients in the modulation of infant sleep: A review of the literature. *Nutritional Neuroscience, 21*(3), 151-161.

37. Bedrosian, T.A., & Nelson, R.J. (2017). Timing of light exposure affects mood and brain circuits. *Translational Psychiatry, 7*(1), e1017.

38. Pandi-Perumal, S.R., Smits, M., Spence, W., Srinivasan, V., Cardinali, D.P., Lowe, A.D., & Kayumov, L. (2007). Dim light melatonin onset (DLMO): a tool for the analysis of circadian phase in human sleep and chronobiological disorders. *Progress in Neuro-Psychopharmacology and Biological Psychiatry, 31*(1), 1-11.

39. Cho, C.H., Lee, H.J., Yoon, H.K., Kang, S.G., Bok, K.N., Jung, K.Y., ... & Lee, E.I. (2016). Exposure to dim artificial light at night increases REM sleep and awakenings in humans. *Chronobiology International, 33*(1), 117-123.

Chapter 11: Managing a sleep crisis with kindness

1. Gerhardt, S. (2014). *Why love matters: How affection shapes a baby's brain.* Routledge.

2. Lupton, D., Pedersen, S., & Thomas, G.M. (2016). Parenting and digital media: from the early web to contemporary digital society. *Sociology Compass, 10*(8), 730-743.

3. Mindell, J.A., Li, A.M., Sadeh, A., Kwon, R., & Goh, D.Y. (2015). Bedtime routines for young children: a dose-dependent association with sleep outcomes. *Sleep, 38*(5), 717-722.

4. Task Force on Sudden Infant Death Syndrome. (2016). SIDS and other sleep-related infant deaths: Updated 2016 recommendations for a safe infant sleeping environment. *Pediatrics, 138*(5), e20162938.

5. Christodulu, K.V., & Durand, V.M. (2004). Reducing bedtime disturbance and night waking using positive bedtime routines and sleep restriction. *Focus on Autism and Other Developmental Disabilities, 19*(3), 130-139.

6. Taylor, D.J., & Roane, B.M. (2010). Treatment of insomnia in adults and children: a practice-friendly review of research. *Journal of Clinical Psychology, 66*(11), 1137-1147.

7. Tzischinsky, O., Shlitner, A., & Lavie, P. (1993). The association between the nocturnal sleep gate and nocturnal onset of urinary 6-sulfatoxymelatonin. *Journal of Biological Rhythms, 8*(3), 199-209.

8. Jenni, O.G., & LeBourgeois, M.K. (2006). Understanding sleep–wake behavior and sleep disorders in children: the value of a model. *Current Opinion in Psychiatry, 19*(3), 282.

9. Field, T. (2017). Infant sleep problems and interventions: A review. *Infant Behavior and Development, 47*, 40-53.

10. Kuypers, L. (2011). *The Zones of Regulation.* San Jose: Think Social Publishing.

11. McDaniel, B.T., & Teti, D.M. (2012). Coparenting quality during the first three months after birth: The role of infant sleep quality. *Journal of Family Psychology, 26*(6), 886.

12. McLeish, J., & Redshaw, M. (2019). 'Being the best person that they can be and the best mum': a qualitative study of community volunteer doula support for disadvantaged mothers before and after birth in England. *BMC pregnancy and childbirth, 19*(1), 21.

13. Tomori, C. (2018). *Changing cultures of night-time breastfeeding and sleep in the US* (pp. 115-30). Bristol, UK: Policy Press.

14. Hookway, L. (2019). *Holistic Sleep Coaching. Gentle Alternatives to Sleep Training for Health and Childcare Professionals.* Praeclarus Press: Amarillo

15. Elrod, H. (2016). *The Miracle Morning: The 6 Habits That Will Transform Your Life Before 8AM: Change your life with one of the world's highest rated self-help books.* Hachette UK.

16. Voltaire, S.T., & Teti, D.M. (2018). Early nighttime parental interventions and infant sleep regulation across the first year. *Sleep medicine, 52*, 107-115.

17. Shubitz, E. (2014). What Is the Ideal Infant Group Care Environment: Montessori Nido versus Infant Daycare Programs. *NAMTA Journal, 39*(2), 149-167.

Chapter 12: Situational sleep stress

1. O'Rourke, M.P., & Spatz, D.L. (2019). Women's Experiences with Tandem Breastfeeding. *MCN: The American Journal of Maternal/Child Nursing, 44*(4), 220-227.

2. Proffit, W.R., & Frazier-Bowers, S.A. (2009). Mechanism and control of tooth eruption: overview and clinical implications. *Orthodontics & craniofacial research, 12*(2), 59-66.

3. Cunha, R.F., Boer, F.A.C., Torriani, D.D., & Frossard, W.T.G. (2001). Natal and neonatal teeth: review of the literature. *Pediatric Dentistry, 23*(2), 158-162.

4. Cheelo, M., Lodge, C.J., Dharmage, S.C., Simpson, J.A., Matheson, M., Heinrich, J., & Lowe, A.J. (2015). Paracetamol exposure in pregnancy and early childhood and development of childhood asthma: a systematic review and meta-analysis. *Archives of Disease in Childhood, 100*(1), 81-89.

5. Massignan, C., Cardoso, M., Porporatti, A.L., Aydinoz, S., Canto, G.D.L., Mezzomo, L.A.M., & Bolan, M. (2016). Signs and symptoms of primary tooth eruption: a meta-analysis. *Pediatrics, 137*(3), e20153501.

Chapter 13: Support yourself to better sleep

1. Taylor, E. (2014). Becoming us: 8 steps to grow a family that thrives. Three Turtles Press.

Index